THE ARTS AND DISABILITIES

THE ARTS
AND
DISABILITIES

*A Creative Response to
Social Handicap*

EDITED BY

GEOFFREY LORD

EDINBURGH:
MACDONALD PUBLISHERS
1981

© Carnegie UK Trust 1981

ISBN 0 904265 62 5 (*cased*)
      0 904265 61 7 (*paper*)

Published by
Macdonald Publishers
Edgefield Road, Loanhead, Midlothian EH20 9SY
for
Carnegie United Kingdom Trust
Comely Park House, Dunfermline, Fife KY12 7EJ

Printed in Great Britain by
Macdonald Printers (Edinburgh) Limited
Edgefield Road, Loanhead, Midlothian EH20 9SY

CONTENTS

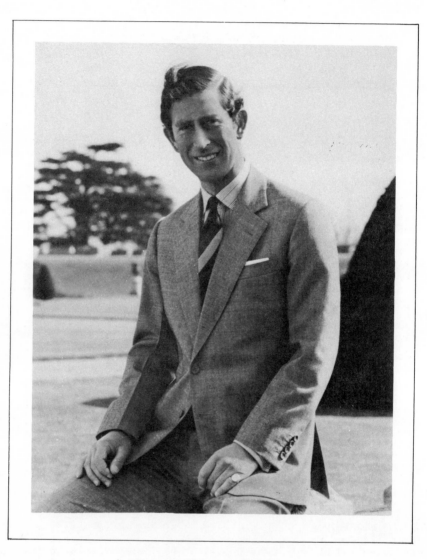

HIS ROYAL HIGHNESS
THE PRINCE OF WALES

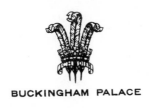

I doubt if many people in Britain realize that there are over three million physically and mentally handicapped people in this country, - in other words, something like 5½% of the population. That is a substantial figure by any standards and of this figure 190,000 are wheelchair cases. I think it would be true to say that there tends to be a deep-seated embarrassment on the part of the able-bodied majority towards the handicapped minority - a natural human reaction towards those who are "different" in some way or other. And yet you only have to visit hospitals, homes or witness paraplegic games, as I do on frequent occasions, to discover that many handicaps are the result of accidents or illness; accidents or illness which could suddenly strike any of us down at any moment.

To me this is a sobering thought, but despite the heartwarming evidence (contained in this book) of the beneficial and psychological effect that the arts can have on the handicapped - both from the therapeutic and emotional standpoint - we still seem incapable of doing enough to make it possible for the handicapped to enjoy the arts and entertainment as much as they would like. Comparisons are invidious, but in America it seems that a more enlightened concern has been shown for the plight of the handicapped than in Britain. For example, any public arts facility, theatre, concert hall, arts centre or museum may jeopardize future government aid if it fails to provide accessibility for all to its presentations or premises.

To my mind, the important point to remember is that all of us, whatever our disability, are given some kind of artistic awareness which enriches our lives. How much more important is it, therefore, to ensure that those who are physically and mentally disabled receive every opportunity to enrich their lives through contact with the arts on as normal a basis as possible. After all, it is only a question of thinking of others as we would hope they would think of us if we were in similar circumstances. This book explains the position far better than I can, so I would recommend turning the page . . .

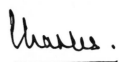

ACKNOWLEDGEMENTS

The Carnegie United Kingdom Trustees wish to acknowledge with sincere thanks the advice, co-operation and help of several individuals and organisations leading to the success of the initial seminars and the production of this book. In particular they wish to thank:

The Scottish Arts Council, and its Director, Timothy Mason, for the joint sponsorship of the Stirling Seminar, and for the generous grant towards the production of this book;

Alexander Dunbar, former Director of the Scottish Arts Council, for his overall guidance;

Professor Henry Walton of Edinburgh who was Chairman at Stirling;

Dr Duncan Guthrie of the Disabilities Study Unit who was Chairman at Dartington;

George Wilson, Director of the Royal Association for Disability and Rehabilitation;

David Dunsmuir, Principal Officer of the Scottish Council for Disability;

Peter Cox, Principal, and staff of the Dartington College of Arts;

Tom Griffiths and staff of the Devon Centre;

Dr W. A. Cramond, Principal and Vice-Chancellor of Stirling University, and his staff;

Rod Fisher, Information Officer of the Arts Council of Great Britain; and especially

The speakers and contributors to this book:

Lynn Eskow, Claudia Flanders, Dorothy Heathcote, Sue Jennings, Pat Keysell, Joyce Laing, Gina Levete, David Mumford, Alastair Pye, Veronica Sherborne, Cherry Vooght, David Ward and colleagues Bruce Kent and Keith Yon;

The reporters: Sue Innes and Bill Seary;

All guest participants; and the staff of Comely Park House for their administrative services.

In the book the word "artists" is used to cover all practitioners in the arts, and words of masculine form are used to cover reference to persons of both sexes.

Introduction

The excellence of every art must consist in the complete accomplishment of its purpose. — Inscription above the entrance to the Victoria and Albert Museum, London.

There is magic in the arts. Anyone who has marvelled at the treasures of Tutankhamun or of Pompeii will never forget their brilliance. Anyone who has been able to attend a Promenade concert, or been thrilled by Oscar Peterson or George Shearing at the piano, or Alan Hacker on clarinet, or Itzhak Perlman on violin, will appreciate the magic. Anyone who has enjoyed and appreciated the humour of Michael Flanders and Donald Swann on stage will remember and be inspired. Those who have been excited by the Beatles or Elton John will remember and may try to emulate them. The memories encourage other interests, other activities and participation.

Many will just enjoy similar performances on radio and television, but for a substantial number of people even this is not possible. The problem of access is but one reason why thousands who are handicapped or disadvantaged can be denied the opportunity and pleasure of appreciating the arts. Those who can enjoy the arts may tend to take them for granted and forget their good fortune.

There is even more magic when talented artists, teachers and tutors employ the arts for the benefit of those with disability. They open up a new dimension in life, a new world for many young and old, yet little is recognised about such work. Behind the magic is much hard work, common sense and a desire to create opportunities for pleasure, enjoyment, education and therapy. Art, drama and speech, mime, movement and music in the hands of gifted and caring practitioners are a force for good.

Because of this belief the Carnegie United Kingdom Trustees initiated a series of residential Seminars to encourage leaders of organisations concerned with disability to review with practitioners the major features of the arts as recreation and as therapy. The first Seminar in 1978 at Dartington College of Arts was an important initiative at a College noted for its pioneering work. The discussions opened many eyes and encouraged guests to share expertise; there was also a little conflict with an awareness of the differing needs and difficulties between recreational, educational and therapeutic aims. The second Seminar at Stirling University was sponsored jointly with the Scottish Arts Council, whose former Director, Alexander Dunbar, and his successor, Timothy Mason, share in the desire for progress in an underdeveloped area of work.

Both Seminars within the theme *The Arts for the benefit and care of disability* were mainly concerned with participatory arts activities and to learn about the role of tutors. The talents of the artists, the caring approach, and the desire to ensure that the handicapped have equal opportunities with others to share in the arts, were the highlights of the formal and informal discussions. The written word may not convey the sincerity and importance of the work or the personalities of the speakers as effectively as the impact of their own presentations, but the articles presented here, as edited versions of the talks, emphasise the talent available for progress. They describe the value of the arts for special needs. All of us have needs: some more special than others. The arts can bring satisfaction if they can be shared; artists and teachers of the arts can be instrumental in helping many including the disabled and disadvantaged to relax, to enjoy, to participate and, where desired, to improve their self-esteem. The arts should be enjoyable and rehabilitative.[1]

The Seminars had a limit in their remit so that painting and sculpture were not included, and physical access to performances was not covered. The opportunities and work for disabled artists is another vast area for inquiry. When there is a concentration of talk on what the able-bodied provide in participatory activities for others who are less fortunate, then there is always a danger of appearing to be patronising in attitude and tone. It is hoped that this has been avoided in the overwhelming desire to record the work which occurs daily with those unfortunately handicapped by sensory, mental or physical disability, whether slight or severe.

There appear to be four categories of work concerned with the arts:

ENTERTAINMENT/RECREATION   EDUCATION
SOCIAL INTERACTION   CLINICAL THERAPY

There is some overlap from one to the other and it is this overlap which occasionally produces difficulties. The articles are not an attempt to identify or analyse these categories, although a seminar for this purpose would be invaluable. Chapters 1 to 9 discuss personal approaches within these categories, with Chapter 10 illustrating one organisation's attempt to provide a service mainly for recreation but assisting with social interaction. It is a fact that there is quite a gap, a difference of opinion, even slight conflict between two distinct developing groups.

Those who encourage the use of arts and artists for the recreation and relaxation of groups of disabled believe that the artists trained in their own particular art form should use their skills in a natural creative process encouraging participation and pleasure. They do not and should not aim deliberately at a process of therapy even though there are undoubted therapeutic spin-offs from many of the activities. The mime artist can for example help the deaf person in communication and to increase self-confidence. Most artists would not be interested in being trained as therapists, preferring to use their skills to entertain and educate, and to benefit individuals whether disabled or not.

Whereas those teachers and tutors of the arts who are interested in a distinctive therapy and aim to make their skills and teaching to be of direct therapeutic benefit to an individual — an attempt at a healing process — are very concerned with the needs of training in therapeutic skills. There is no doubt that anyone using the arts as therapy, for example for the mentally ill or disturbed person, should be trained adequately and recognise standards for this process. Equally there is no doubt that a teacher or artist not trained as a therapist should not attempt interpretation or counselling of a personal nature to an individual or group.

Unfortunately there is a grey area — perhaps occupied by the temporarily depressed person or the mentally handicapped person, or an individual suffering from an addiction — which defies normal rules. The arts should be available and of benefit to them and it is important that common sense should be used in establishing any arts activity, for example in the use of dance and movement with the mentally handicapped. The promoter has a responsibility to ensure that the qualifications of the artists/tutors, and the aims and practice of the activity, are examined with the managers of the project whether in a residential or day setting.

The differences of opinion and conflict between the groups are no bad thing, for they ensure examination of aims. Both groups are concerned genuinely with the need for and the provision of high standards in work with the disabled. An important factor therefore is to ensure communication and dialogue about the aims and activities between the different groups, but unfortunately at the present time this does not occur sufficiently. Chapter 11 offers a timely reminder about training for any therapeutic work.

The Carnegie Trustees have been privileged in recent years to be associated with some fine schemes in the development of participatory arts. These include assistance to the late Philip Bailey of Liverpool who investigated the adaptation of musical instruments and music for physically handicapped children, and published his book *They Can Make Music.*[2] In addition the Trustees inaugurated and financed the Drama Board from 1948 to 1979 leading to the ADB examinations now supported by the Department of Education and Science. There is a special qualification for tutors, who may themselves be disabled, to become skilled in work with the disabled. Further support followed to the Dartington College of Arts experiments with the publication of *Hearts and Hands and Voices*[3]; Effective Speech Courses with the National Federation of Women's Institutes and more recently with the National Institute of Adult Education; Drama with the Blind courses; workshops by the Interim Theatre Company and the Scottish Mime Theatre, and the progress of Shape nationally. These projects, some of which are described later, provide a basis for learning. The Seminars commence the wider exchange of experience and expertise.

The purpose of this book is to encourage the reader to learn of some of the opportunities and of the problems, and of the skilled work in the pursuit of excellence. This pursuit is no less evident in work by and with the disabled than in any public performance enjoyed by the masses. It is our hope that as the masses advance there will be more inquiry into the purpose and values of activities in the arts by and for the disabled, with the creation of more and better opportunities in participatory arts.

REFERENCES
1. *The Healing Role of the Arts.* The Rockefeller Foundation, 1978.
2. *They Can Make Music.* Philip Bailey. Oxford University Press, 1973.
3. *Hearts and Hands and Voices.* David Ward. Oxford University Press, 1976.

1

The Therapeutic Aspects of Arts Centres

JOYCE LAING

Q. *Art is an important medium of expression especially for pleasure and relaxation. Yet its value as a therapy is only just beginning to be understood. How do you see its role?*

Before describing and illustrating the uses of art as a form of psychotherapy, I think it would be useful to consider the social situation of today and more importantly of tomorrow, with particular reference to the emotional, mental and spiritual needs of people.

I believe that in the next twenty years arts centres will be in a position to offer as much help, through promotion of the arts and artistic activities, to the psychological well-being of people as did psycho-analytically oriented centres and their consequent influence on society at the end of the last century, or the introduction of the concept of therapeutic communities in the middle of this century.

There is today an avid seeking for a meaningful philosophy of life. People seem to be searching for an identity, the return to a oneness with nature, a coming closer to basic materials and no longer seeing mass production as the answer to everything. It is interesting to note that every autumn for the past few years queues have formed to gain admission to evening classes at the Colleges of Art. Summer schools providing courses in the arts have become similarly popular. Galleries and museums are increasingly visited, especially when there is a participatory role for the audience. Other forms of community experience are also attracting attention: groups which encounter, groups which meditate, workshops in a variety of media and newly formed communities and sects are springing up all over. To understand these new trends and foresee future patterns it is necessary to look at the ever changing patterns of human behaviour throughout history. The aspirations and desires of people, the stresses and illnesses which befall them, are integrally linked to the social conditions and patterns of the age in which we live.

From the beginning of time people's well-being and the arts have been interwoven. From the earliest known times the obtaining of food and shelter must have dictated the total life style. The graphic illustrations by cave-dwellers reflect their needs, and while the material acquisition of food by hunting wild animals was all important, their beliefs focused on the spiritual, the supernatural and the magical to attain these needs. The recent television documentary filming the group of young people who have been attempting to simulate the lives of the Iron Age villagers served to illustrate that their stresses came from the constant struggle to keep warm and finding enough food to eat. However, the knowledge of both performer and viewer that antibiotics, for example, could be immediately available if the demand arose, negated any sense of the historical emotional stresses the early settlers must have experienced.

The priest, the artist and the medicine man have been closely linked throughout history, often being one and the same person, their role being an answer to the emotional needs of the time. And if placating one's mentor offered a feeling of security through the belief that there would be food, shelter and safety, then there could be no more meaningful activity. The patterns of behaviour, which now seem quite bizarre to us, incorporating dance, music and body painting, were inbuilt safety factors not so different from our present-day use of insurance companies and investment! The art form of any age reveals the most deeply held beliefs and spiritual needs of the people of that time. Such examples as the pyramids and tomb sculptures of Egypt, where the people believed in the divinity of their king, shows how a whole culture built up around this creed. The ancient Egyptians believed that their god had substituted his divine being for human form in the being of a king and when the king died his soul continued to live beside the body; thus great care was taken to mummify the body and to encase it with the use of precious metals and gems. From the wall paintings of the tombs we can see that great importance was given not only to the art of embalming but also to the craftsmanship of the funerary offerings which were made for eternity. Healing by touch, by faith, may be as old as mankind but it is from the life of Christ and subsequently from the work of his apostles and followers that we see the miraculous cures through faith healing. Christ practised healing by laying his hands on the sufferer or touching the diseased part of the body or simply raising his hand as if in blessing. There is also the story of a woman who gained recovery from her illness because she touched the hem of Christ's garment, and her act of faith was recognised by Christ.

In faith healing supernatural powers are given to the healer in the eyes of the believer. It is essential the sufferer has faith in the cure and the healer is either the embodiment of a divine being or a person acting as a medium for the divine power.

The art of each period reflects the life-style and beliefs of that time. Anyone interested in Victoriana has at their fingertips a social history of the latter half of the last century. Victorian jewellery in particular seems to encompass the essence of the age. In a time when the possible death of a loved one was an ever present threat, hair lockets and hair rings became high fashion. These tiny mementoes in which a fragment of the hair of the beloved dead one was intricately woven, would be set in the finest gold setting the mourner could afford. Another jewellery fashion, jet necklaces and name brooches, also indicated the loss of a near relative. Fashion too is a fine mirror of social conditions. Relatively young Victorian women could be seen dressed totally in black — a mark of respect for a dead relative — and for widows, black clothing would remain the only acceptable colour for the rest of their days.

Art and fashion are ever changing, but the patterns of health and illness change too, perhaps never more spectacularly than today. For thousands of years medicine has been seen as the hand of power giving the magic potion to the unfortunate sufferer. The healer has given charms, performed magical rites, called upon supernatural powers, brewed concoctions, and now the cures come in tablet form. For the client, often suffering pain, there is little choice — he is obliged to believe.

Q.   *How do these theories fit the practicalities of today?*

Today we live in an age of ever increasing change at an ever increasing speed. Infant mortality is at an all time low and life expectancy has doubled in the last hundred years. Barring accidents we can look forward to our three score years and ten; many will live longer. Consider the disappearing diseases — tuberculosis, although not eradicated, is no longer the fearful ailment as recalled in the vivid paintings of Edvard Munch whose family was ridden with the disease. Pneumonia with its dreaded crisis is now a treatable fever with few dangers. Cholera, diphtheria, poliomyelitis have happily lost their terror. The whole pattern of illness is changing. Many of the present diseases are caused by man-made substances such as pesticides and chemicals and by our own affluence when food, cigarettes and alcohol are readily available to all of us. Not only are cancers, coronary and artery diseases increasing but also the stress illnesses: anxiety, depression, alcoholism, drug addiction. It is a society which has largely solved the problems of poverty, overwork and

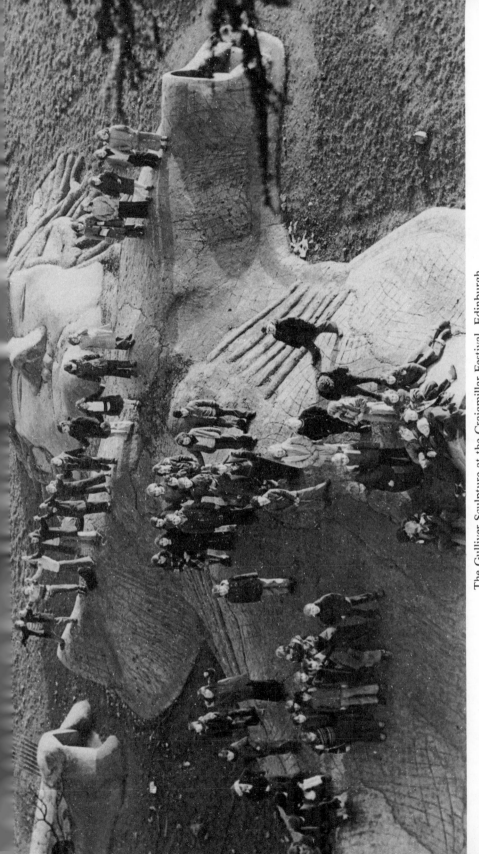

The Gulliver Sculpture at the Craigmillar Festival, Edinburgh

Photos by John Brown

premature death, yet it has created its own problems. There is an urgent search for meaning to replace disintegrating values, for a sense of work in face of redundancy and unemployment, for stable relationships in a breakdown of the family. It would seem then that the future holds a decrease in infectious diseases and a speed of recovery of surgery and convalescence, yet an increase in psychological disorders and all that that implies, such as more crime, more drug abuse, more alcoholism as well as increase in the stress illnesses.

One of the most interesting new social patterns is the involvement by communities in running their own affairs. Disillusioned by waiting for figureheads in central government to solve difficulties, various groups of ordinary people have come together and acted together in the management of community affairs. Craigmillar in Edinburgh is a fine example of this, and interestingly the coming together of the community representatives was not premeditated to work out or manage their own policies in respect to everyday living matters; it happened as the result of a few creative thinkers initiating a community arts festival. That may seem a lucky coincidence to some; I prefer to believe that the desire for a community arts festival was the unconscious wish of the people to reassert their identity and value, to make decisions and to organise their own lives. So we see another factor emerging—the inner resources of people.

A detail from the Gulliver Sculpture

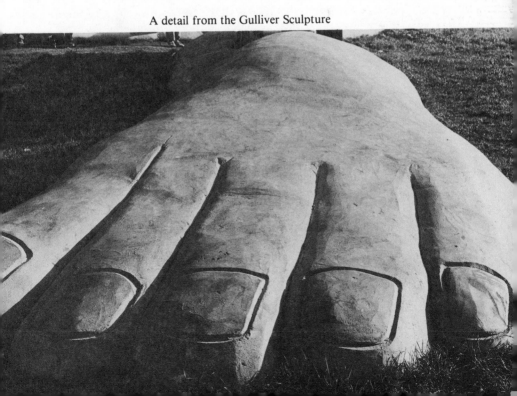

Q. *Can these human inner resources be tapped through the arts?*

Access to inner resources taps the same process as any creative activity. Thus the queues at the Art Colleges, the reawakening of old crafts, the enthusiasm to join groups may be viewed not as inexplicable phenomena but as a balancing of society's psyche in order to achieve stability in our lives. Yet art is still considered by many as only pictures in frames to be hung in galleries. Art is much bigger than that. The true art of today will be the art which answers emotional needs and seeks alternative thinking to problems. We need the artists, the inventors, the initiators, the creative among us to give expression to our unconscious wishes and to explore solutions to our fears. It is difficult for us to see the art of our age in perspective because we are too close to it. We can, however, see the tendencies and inclinations. Art has never been so diverse: there is at the same time a keen interest in conservation and respect for the craftsmanship of the past, and a tremendous advancement in art techniques such as kinetics, electronics and laser. There is a re-awareness of the spiritual quality of life compared to the materialistic inclinations of the past decades.

The growth of arts centres symbolises the needs of society today. People are beginning to look at their own inner resources to solve their problems and enrich their lives. With encouragement, stimulus and support, and in the right milieu, they can tap their own creativity and develop their appreciation and understanding of others.

No-one can predict what will happen in the next decade; however, many of the trends are obvious. It is certain there will be more leisure time for all, earlier retirement and possibly further unemployment. The cost of keeping a patient in hospital, a child in residential care or a person in prison will increase to the extent that the country will be forced to look at alternatives. Day centre resources both in care for disabilities and in being the hub of each community's social life are a viable alternative. Arts centres then are placed in a highly responsible position for they can offer, if they develop their resources, some of the answers to these trends.

Q. *What about the needs of patients and help through treatment?*

There will be two main groups of people seeking treatment or therapy. There will be people who are suffering from a definable illness and who can appropriately be referred to a hospital or clinic and treated by known and proven methods, and there will be the people who are seeking meaning in their lives and solutions to inner disturbance. Many in the latter group may find that activities offered through the arts may help them to resolve their situation. Also most illnesses are fortunately transitory and in-patient treatment may only be needed for a short time. Furthermore, if the type of day centre resources were available they might provide preventative as well as supportive measures, thus evading the need for hospitalisation for certain psychological conditions.

To my knowledge, all the drama, dance, mime workshops for children, and Saturday art classes for children at art colleges, and music and pop evenings are oversubscribed. Perhaps if more of these stimulating and genuinely educational activities were offered to children there would be fewer truants and the consequent children in trouble.

By looking now at the uses of art therapy in treating people who are ill, it is possible to see how the arts can be used by anyone. Illness and health after all are not black and white aspects of life. Art, like dreams, is not solely the prerogative of the ill or disturbed. Art is a hot-line with the unconscious and it is from the unconscious that the clues of the origin of problems emerge. In art therapy, then, patients' art is a transmission, often unconscious, of the inner self. For some patients, their paintings or other created objects are the only perceptible means of communication of their inner struggle for health. Although the patient may not understand the content of his art work he will have deeply rooted feelings about it and will only allow it to be seen by an artist who understands the language of imagery. The feelings expressed could not have been put into words, yet the significance of the images unfold little by little, clarifying the underlying problems. It is only within the relationship of partnership, which the art therapist will have established with the patient, that some of the sources of the problems will become apparent. As the patient's self-discovery continues, self-growth, self-confidence and self-healing take place.

If art centres are to become resources for the well-being of the whole community then they must develop with the understanding of the psychological needs of society today.

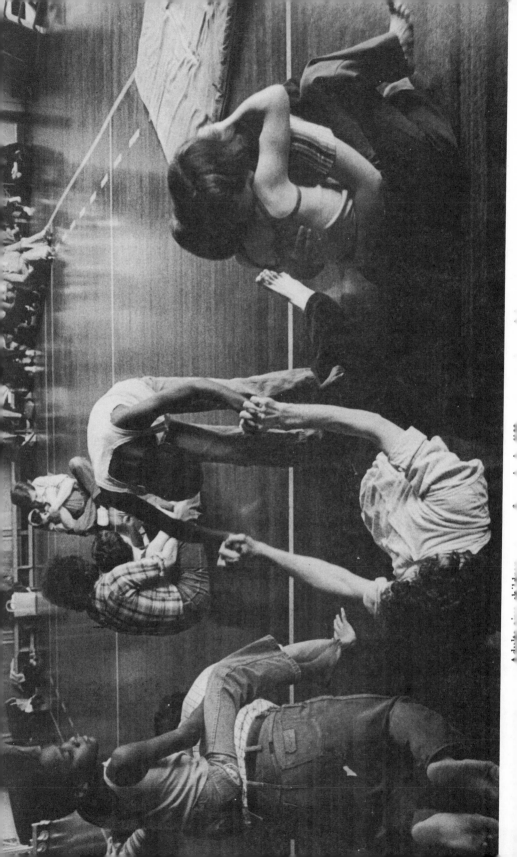

2

A Sense of Movement

VERONICA SHERBORNE

Q. *Your excellent film is very concerned with movement, or even what many inexperienced people
might think of as a form of physical education
rather than a particular art form. How is movement
used with the disabled and why did you make the
film?*

I made the film *A Sense of Movement* in order to show how certain
movement experiences can contribute to the development of children
who are severely mentally handicapped. I worked with a former student,
John Cannon, in a Bristol ESN(S) school and the film shows him
teaching a class of 5 to 8-year-old children and a class of 14 to 16-year-
olds. The film was made by postgraduate students in the Department of
Drama of the University of Bristol, and we spent five Wednesday
afternoons filming half-hour lessons with each class.

The film shows progression in the building of relationships. Children
in the younger class, who are functioning at about the age of normal
children of 18 months to 2½ years, begin by being mainly passive
recipients of movement experiences. The teacher involves teacher's aides,
senior children in the school and a secondary school boy as partners for
the younger children. The adults and adolescents give the young children
the experience of being supported and contained in different ways, which
"feeds in" confidence and security to the children.

From this basis the next stage, which is a significant one, can develop.
The children begin to take responsibility for moving the adults and start
to interact with the adult in shared movement play; a 50-50 relationship
develops.

The children having enjoyed relating and interacting with an adult are
now ready for the next stage, which is to work with another child, and we
can see the beginnings of relationships with a child partner.

Children in the senior class related well to a partner except for three particularly retarded children who had adult or adolescent partners. During the five weeks of filming the senior children progressed from partner work to working in threes and fours, and eventually succeeded in working together as a whole group of 12 children with their teacher, teacher's aide and the schoolboy.

Progression was also seen in the different kinds of relationship play. The younger children can cope with the simplest forms of partner play and these are developed further by the older children. I call these "with" relationships where the child co-operates with a partner and can support, contain, and care for another person. The older children are introduced to relationships "against" a partner, in which a child can test the firmness, steadiness and strength of a partner. Through this kind of partner-play the children learn to organise and control their energy and to direct and focus their strength. The artist as therapist works to allow the disabled person to participate in the art form. Some of the older children are successful in both "with" and "against" activities, and can let go of the weight of their bodies, and can concentrate and use their strength in a positive way.

Q.   *You rightly emphasise the development of relation-*
     ships and there is also encouragement of touch.
     How does this help?

While the children are being extended in terms of making relationships, the movement programme is also developing the children's awareness of their bodies. The emphasis for the younger children is on awareness of the body as a whole in different ground-based activities such as rolling and sliding, and in activities such as somersaulting over the adult's shoulder, and being contained and rocked. The young children are then helped to become aware of their hips, knees and feet. It is extremely important that severely retarded children should experience and learn to control the weight-bearing parts of the body as this will help them to move about as normally as possible. This awareness is built up first from sitting, without bearing weight, and then developed into activities such as jumping and falling.

The senior children extend the awareness of their knees and the control of the weight of the body in activities such as jumping, landing, and being stable and firm. The teacher also "feeds in" for the older children that they have a trunk, a centre, by making them more aware of their backs, stomachs, hips and shoulders. This is often best experienced

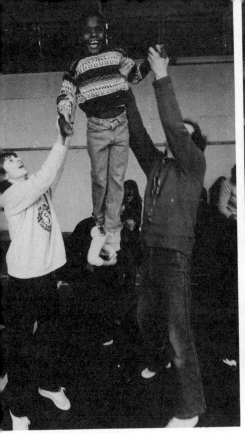

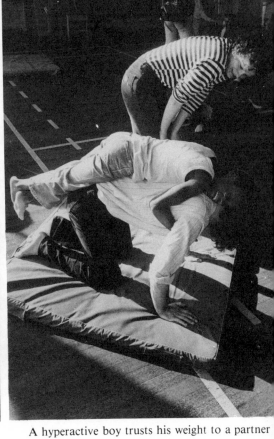

ng supported by two people is much enjoyed   A hyperactive boy trusts his weight to a partner

Photos by Clive Landen

A tense disturbed boy allows himself to be carried by two adults

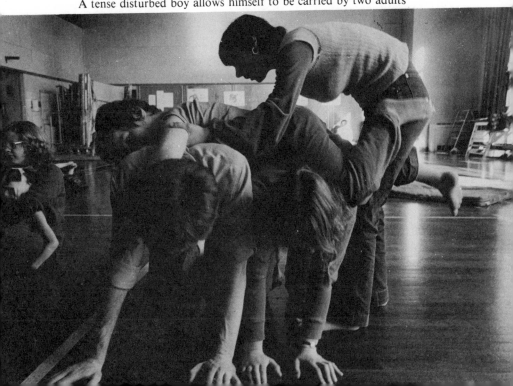

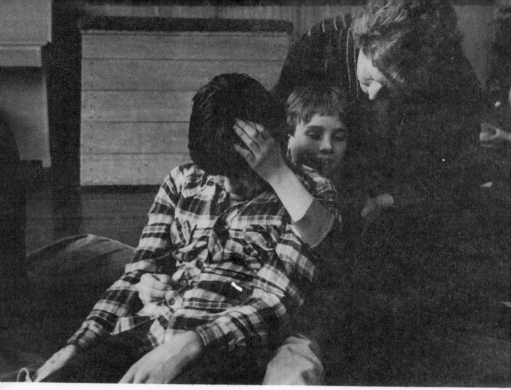

A boy with autistic tendencies can "look after" his partner but will not look at what he is doing

Photos by Clive Landen

A quiet ending with cradling and singing

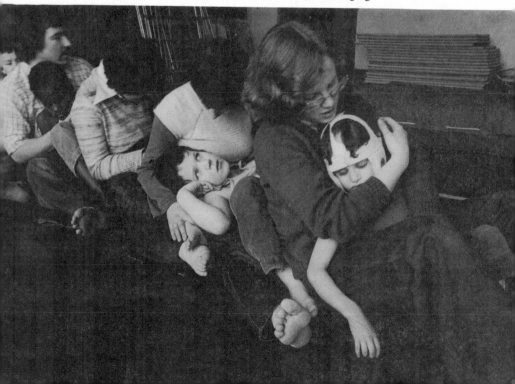

against the ground, on large apparatus, or against other people. A great deal of body awareness has to be fed in through tactile experiences. Children who have some feeling for the middle of their body can curl up in a tight ball and can resist efforts to open them out. Children need to be aware of their centre as this makes an essential link between their head and their feet which helps them to move in an integrated connected way.

A movement lesson may be carefully planned and presented as a series of exercises, but the best lessons are those which grow from what happens in the class. The teacher observes the children's efforts and uses some of their ideas to develop his lesson. With experience a teacher can build a lesson combining children's contributions with the introduction of new experiences which are relevant to the children's level of development and which will extend them.

The movement lesson should be enjoyed by the teacher and helpers as much as by the children. The teacher ensures that all the children are successful and develops their potential as fully as possible.

REFERENCES

Physical and Creative Activities for Mentally Handicapped Children. Editor, C. Upton. Cambridge University Press, 1979. Three chapters including "Content of a developmental movement programme."

Physical Education for Children with Special Needs. Editor, L. Groves. Cambridge University Press, 1979. One chapter on building relationships through movement.

FILMS*

In Touch, movement for mentally handicapped children, 1965.

Explorations, movement for drama, 1971.

A Sense of Movement, movement for mentally handicapped children, 1976 (selected in 1978 for preservation by the National Film Archives).

*The films are distributed and available on loan from Concord Films Council, 201 Felixstowe Road, Ipswich, Suffolk.

3

Talking with Confidence

CHERRY VOOGHT

Q. *You seem to have developed a unique style of group work with those who are shy, anxious, very lacking in confidence, or inhibited in a stressful way. What is the background and aim?*

There is an apparent arrogance in the title of the courses. It bears no relevance whatever to my state of mind in preparing this address.

I am aware too that most of the readers will be specialists dealing with the varied physical and mental problems that flesh is heir to. You are more fortunate than you perhaps realise. I have spent the last decade or so working with people who think they are normal. Furthermore we think we know what "normal" means. I wonder if any thinking person would care to define "normal" in terms of a human being?

I have worked in very varied areas during this time; a great deal of the work has been with Women's Institute groups, but I have also worked on these experimental courses with local education authority groups open to all through newspaper advertisement. The main attraction seems to be the word "confidence," and among the participants who come to work with me for two or three days there are inevitably one or two who are hoping for divine intervention to perform a miracle. As a teacher I have found myself in an Autolycus situation — "a snapper-up of unconsidered trifles" — for, in human terms, that is what many of my "normal" students have shown themselves to be. And it is only with patience, constant reassurance and praise over the smallest achievement that they begin to realise something of their own potential.

The courses I lead now have the name *Talking with Confidence*.[1] It is not a good name, but it is better than a former one — *Effective Speech*. In working with the BBC, the first name suggested was *Thinking and Speaking* and later courses were featured under the *Wordpower* series.

All these titles lean too heavily on the end product—words/speech. The essence of the work is concerned with human relationships, and that much-abused word "communication," often tossed about so lightly by those who seem to know little about it in human terms.

The following extract is the opening of a paper I wrote in 1977 for the Carnegie UK Trust which supported the early work:

"The essence of education is the transmission of what we have discovered."
— Jerome S. Bruner, *The Relevance of Education*, 1972

These words concisely sum up the concept and belief on which I have based this method of teaching. I have been free to think anew, and to rediscover the implications of the varied aspects of my professional work—and finally to bring them together into a pattern which can be passed on to help other people to rediscover themselves and their potential.

The great stumbling-block to human progress is lack of confidence, of being unable to trust oneself and other people. Today's life-atmosphere of pessimism, fear and suspicion is creating more and more problems for already insecure people, so the emphasis of the courses has essentially been on the positive and optimistic, the rebuilding of trust in oneself and other people, and in life itself. During the seven years of development I have taught several hundred students of both sexes, in small groups totally varied in age, physical ability and background. From this experience I draw this conclusion with utter conviction—that if you can encourage, even cherish a student throughout a practical experience of happy, positive and profound thought, you can give them the power to reverse the negative trend and to go forward—and on and on. The gift of speech and the ability to communicate are then rooted and lasting.

So that is what the courses aim to do; to persuade the student to trust himself and other people in an insecure and untrusting world; to accept himself as he is and make the very best of it; and to realise that

"I do not like the human race,
I do not like its silly face."

is a hopeless philosophy by which to live. If he can be assured that as himself he has something special to give, and receive, it is a new beginning, and he will find the courage to opt out of the rat-race, materially or psychologically, of trying to keep up with the Joneses.

Very few of the students could be regarded as "sick" in strictly medical terms, but if there is even a remote possibility then the priority is to persuade them to get specialist help. They are generally vaguely-anxious, unhappy people, feeling themselves to be inadequate, and wanting to do something about it. A few of the students who arrive to share the courses are easily identified as handicapped in some way.

Many are less easy to recognise since we cannot see the mind-locked fears which deaden their lives.

> "As I was going down the stair
> I met a man who wasn't there.
> He wasn't there again today.
> I wish, I wish he'd go away."

Q.   *How do you structure your courses for the range of personalities and difficulties you must encounter?*

Throughout the courses I try to use a very down-to-earth and practical approach—to reassure and to help the students to accept work which is quite outside their normal experience. From the beginning there must be a "family" feeling with an atmosphere of fun and enjoyment and absolutely no critical attitudes.

This allows hard work and serious thinking to be possible when the students develop naturally during the progress of the course. Movement has an important part to play—not only to relieve tension but as a practical exploration of person-to-person communication. Trust and mutual-dependence exercises are also key factors in the beginning processes. At every stage there is very full discussion and analysis of the discoveries made, and this is a natural and logical way-in to the growth of language. Personal achievement is built in step by step—through improvisation, simulation, role-playing, poetry-reading and writing, and finally through the formal techniques of public speaking.

There is never any real off-duty time—evening recreation sessions keep the group together sharing games, dancing, singing, reading and recounting—anything that creates participation, fun, conversation and, above all, laughter—which I believe to be the greatest therapy of all and a powerful force in education. Experience has served to strengthen my belief that you cannot teach anybody anything, you can only make it possible for them to learn.

There are no concessions made in the work-plan. It is the same for all, and each student is free to join in at his own level, whatever the age, background, physical and mental capacity. The practical and psychological results are always striking, sometimes astonishing, especially with apparent non-starters. They are also lasting, and I have watched many individuals go from strength to strength over the years. For many too it has meant the end of loneliness in the enduring friendships they have made. They come to the follow-on courses to be encouraged to grow even further, and for the fun and the companionship.

The important thing we should all surely realise from experience is not how different are the needs of the people we try to help, but how much alike. Reassurance, companionship, fun and recreation, human contact, strong and caring leadership—these are common denominator needs with all the disadvantaged people I have met, and many of the so-called "normal." Perhaps we all tend to have a "little boxes" attitude to our own area of work—to be over-protective, even over-possessive concerning our special territory. If we had more opportunity, and the will, to share our experiences more fully we might defy the law of mathematics and find that $2 + 2 + 2 + 2$ equals more than 8.

Q. *What are your views about the needs in teaching and leadership for the use of drama as a main instrument in courses?*

Between previous and present visits to Dartington there has stretched for me a long, hard road of discovery—in trying to find some answers between the one extreme and the other of what drama can mean. From the experiences of this journey I would encourage consideration of the following points:

1. As I have been so concerned with teacher-training in the past years my first point is almost inevitably concerned with the training of teachers who use drama for educational purposes, whether for the "normal," or for any therapeutic purpose. Indeed I would go so far as to say that *any* use of drama can and should be therapeutic if we can accept the definition

    "Concerned with the art of healing and the improvement of physical and mental condition."

If we, as teachers, can so affect human lives, then surely our experience must be thorough and widely-based. Good drama work needs a good drama teacher, who could if necessary cope with a varied range of classes. This must be even more important when the teacher is dealing with the more fragile human mind or body; it is simply not enough to add superficial drama skills to medical knowledge of a condition, or superficial medical knowledge to the most expert drama skills.

I use the term "widely-based" because I feel that we should recognise that we may all have too limited a vision, that we do not look far enough to the left and right of the disability which is our special concern. This is understandable when one thinks of the energy and concentration needed. But there is a danger of our becoming speed readers of humanity, concentrating on our particular centre of the human page, which may give us a lot of information but denies us the opportunity to make full use of it. We know too little about what the rest are doing.

2. I am sure that in the teaching of physically or mentally handicapped people we must always keep an eye on our own attitude and involvement. Even the best teachers cannot always avoid the danger of becoming too intensive, obsessive, uptight and over-anxious. But we need commitment and not obsession for the sake of those we lead.

   We cannot be unaware that drama teaching can attract well-meaning but inadequate craftsmen who simply do not recognise that it is far too easy to use students as guinea-pigs on whom to work out one's own personal problems, rather than vice versa. As an examiner I have seen too many sessions which are self-indulgent and meaningless, and sometimes could be very aptly described as "erotic writhings in a splash of magenta." Our work must often take our students on imaginative flights — this is their need — but I am sure that it is equally important that we return them solidly to earth. Everything we do must have a clear common-sense purpose — not merely processes, but progress.

3. In the choice and training of leaders to work with disadvantaged people I believe that life-experience and personality are more important than academic achievement. Sensitivity, affection and compassion are the essential foundations on which to build the technical skills.

4. In recognising the need for more suitable support-workers to share the work of the drama teacher, I think we could make more definite approaches to reputable national organisations, to enlist mature, caring and reliable people as practical workers and organisers. It may even be possible to think of minimal payment, since so many would be glad to increase small incomes — and would like to put things on a regular business footing. Similarly we should never underestimate the value of residential courses, with their off-duty social time.

5. I confess to being worried by the growth of labels over the past years, which can provide an open invitation for unsuitable people to jump on the bandwagon of leadership. Encounter groups, T groups, psycho-drama — we must be sure that we know what they really mean, and what we are doing. Mystique can be a splendid defence-mechanism. I once joined a so-called encounter group in an effort to see whether they could help in Samaritan work. A very early session was given to what I can only call "childhood dissection," and when our leader learned that my father had died when I was six months old, and that my only and older brother had died in a motor accident at the age of twenty-seven, he almost gleefully welcomed me as a natural disaster and assured me that "my life would inevitably be concentrated on a permanent search for a father." As I was by then Adviser to the National Federation of Women's Institutes I felt I must have missed my way somewhere.

I am sure that leadership must be positive and cheerful — for as I have said, there is nothing more valuable than laughter. I believe in relaxation and trust and enjoyment, not in morbid and almost competitive soul-stripping. In the right atmosphere problems will emerge naturally and undramatically, and are then received in the same quiet way. This in itself is reassuring and healing.

6. My final point really looks back to where I began. I am sure everyone must recognise the importance of preventive work, especially the provision of courses for "normal" people in which those under stress can find refuge and a new and lasting beginning. Let us learn to assist with problems before they magnify into complete breakdown needing prolonged remedial help.

REFERENCE

1. *Talking with Confidence* was recorded by Westward TV and a 30 minute video cassette of this work is available on loan from the Carnegie UK Trust office.

4

Drama and the Mentally Handicapped

DOROTHY HEATHCOTE

Q. *You often state in articles that you are an amateur.*
    Why, when you are undoubtedly an expert in drama
    as education?

Come, share in a situation with me: a visiting teacher working in a
hospital for handicapped people. Nurse watching. On the floor, a large
man dressed in a furry costume. Children gathered round trying to
"mend a paw" with a large bandage.

Nurse: "But if he's supposed to be a proper dog, why does he have to
have one big red velvet ear? And why not two, then they could match?"
This is the kind of question that I keep trying to answer.

My biggest problem in teaching is that I am an amateur! No college of
education or university department ever found me inside their august
portals until I entered them as a lecturer appointed to teach others to
teach. So, as an amateur I tend to use common sense. Not that I am
against academic study or theories, but those addicted to this form of
knowing do tend to discount common sense as being "hunch" and
written-down words as "proper knowledge."

The real problem of learning and teaching is really the difference
between knowing something yourself, and trying to use it in such a way
that other people are inducted into knowing. My areas of knowing and
teaching are applied in "people" situations, and if you are a doctor
reading this you know the problems of people, because people are
"varmints" and won't fit into nicely pre-packaged ideas. The skills of
teaching are the skills of interaction, perception and of paying close
attention to signals; to learn this one has to remain curious, take risks
and watch outcomes with a keen eye and systems of appraisal and, above
all, we have to remain enthusiastic in the face of much doubt. This is

because, in our culture, examination is often the respectable and safe way of testing ideas.

Q. *What is the main message of your film* Albert *that you are trying to convey?*

Albert develops the situation of a poor lonely man at first hidden in a corner of a room by newspapers, who when approached by children registers fear and apprehension. Perhaps some of the children feel a little like this or recognise the anxiety in the person? Soon they encourage him to talk and want to help him. The film shows how natural emotions come into play and focus into a learning situation, where the children can question what to do and why.

What happens in the situation must be experienced in reality by them — I never ask them consciously to pretend.

To keep this reality I try to make something occur to which they only have to respond. These occurrences must really happen, for example a person may be there to meet them. A thing needing to be done might be there plainly demonstrating what needs doing. A combination of both may be there.

The occurrence or person must be very clearly defined — one of the methods I use often is to create a bizarre or noticeable provocation so that no-one can miss it — it can intrude on their vision, their space: a gentle invasion, but inexorable nevertheless and capable of constant development.

To achieve this, I tend to look to "epic" materials for my provocations. Epic material bypasses "little jobs" and reaches first for relationships, out of which working together can begin. The basis of epic material lies in these areas: striving, feeling, great fearing, joy, labour, painful trials, carrying heavy responsibility, or celebrating.

The occurrence or meeting must demonstrate the need to take decisions. Each decision must be the choice of the group, using their information, their expertise, their choice: as in *Albert*, where the group questioned whether they should take the man to school or to home, and decided to check with the Headmistress, and so their direct involvement in decision-taking began.

Q. *If decisions can be made, how do you recognise progress in an individual or group?*

Each decision is a learning process and must be tested in outcome, by the demonstration of that outcome leading to further decisions being taken.

Progression for me lies in important signs and facts:

1. The children or adults anticipate the presence of the "role" or event more and more.
2. They recall and recount it and their part in it afterwards and between meetings.
3. They take power over or within the events.
4. They show opinion and stick to it, thinking around it more and more.
5. There is language flow and expression demonstrated which break into new language patterns, or change in physical demeanour.
6. Concentration begins to show intensity but openness to others.

Obviously progress is often hidden because of language, and often physical damage is gross, but a new eyelid flutter, a new sound is a miracle of achievement.

I use theatre forms to declare problems and reveal choices, and I am always highly selective in how I present the material, especially in use of language, stance and heights. I use no "canned" effects. For music any instrument is suitable where people can be seen playing it, and I try to bring these instruments to the group members also, so that they may try them. Portable instruments are preferred to the piano, such as violin, flute, oboe, guitar. These latter are essentially sociable in that the player can have strong eye contact with the group.

All ideas must develop slowly, keeping high energy but slow pace, with time for experience, expression of response, adjustment of attitude and developing a sense of "where we're at."

Leaders must put aside pre-knowing so as to avoid taking decisions away from the group. All other logic must be encountered and used, and this means a high toleration of ambiguity.

The word "drama" is a blanket word which has many manifestations. Usually people have a mental image in their minds of "a re-enactment of a situation, done in public, by people, while others watch." But when you think of that it is also true of church services, and performing magicians, and "people who bring their harps to parties." In its widest interpretation it simply means that we can, by a shift in the head, experience an "as if it were" reality, and for the time perceive it as the real world. We do it when we read of others and think inside their situation, instead of about their situation. We do it when we conjure a world in advance of the real experience — before a driving test or interview which will matter to us; we do it when we relive an experience afterwards to mull it over. So, at one end of the scale of interpretations we have theatrical performances of great complexity, while at the other end we have this very private exploration.

The value in the "as if it were" experience is that we can be relieved of the burden of the future, except when we are pre-living a situation which inexorably will come. But even in that situation, we can tentatively experiment with a variety of approaches and outcomes. So dramatic activity, of whatever kind, can be said to provide us with metaphors to our real lives, which in turn allow us to reflect about life's experiences.

Q. *Is this type of dramatic activity not too unreal to help with improvement in daily functioning?*

No, the problems start when others think that the "as if" world is a pretend world, leading us to unreality. In fact it is just the opposite of this. When we reflect on our worlds, even if we indulge in fantasy and stage farces, we are inexorably led eventually to real events, because drama always must deal with the affairs of mankind — even when they are clothed in animal manifestations, or wizards and witches. Which brings me to the brown dog with red velvet ears. The outer form looks silly and "pretend," but in fact the velvet ear is to provide a cuddly feeling, a focus for those who do not see well and a less frightening aspect for the timid — because our dog is a "service agent" for experiences — big enough to ride on, tough enough to fight with you if you want to get rough, and timid when required — if you are ready to learn about caring and tenderness. He is also capable of being very tough with you, if you are ready to learn about handling anger in yourself.

The mystery for me lies in the slow exploration of how we can structure "as if" situations, in order to give a programmed series of experiences which stretch the mentally handicapped in positive and useful ways, for their practical lives and for their inner imaginative lives. How far is it possible for such a person to share in an experience and reflect upon it, because that event has, unlike the experiences of life which are largely chance, been introduced into their experience in a timely way? All too often when drama is used with slow learners, it is used as a "task level" thing where events are simulated but not really explored, where stories are hurried through but not experienced; and yet I have evidence of some rather earth-shattering explorations which seem almost to be Jungian in their manifestation. As if myth were tapped and universals perceived during the action!

Derek and Jim, two 40-year-olds in a villa were looking after me, "as if" I was their mother. They were obviously taking great pleasure from deciding where my chair should be placed in relation to the sunshine which was pouring into the room. They then decided to take me for a run in the car (two chairs, but a very "real" car) to the seaside. Once by the sea they pondered with me about "where the sea comes from." I stimulated this by asking the question (though it reads like a statement), "I've never understood why God made sand." Derek immediately answered, "For the sea to be on top of," but as we continued, we found ourselves discussing "this side" and "the other side" which I began to realise was an exploration of before being born and dying. The whole discussion, however, was also an exploration of children in relation to their parents. They were assuring me that they would look after me until my death, while worrying in a way that they might not be able to manage without me. They also wondered "how old you are when you're born": Jim being of the opinion that you have to be five before you are born, while Derek thought "a bit younger." All of this is in a musing fashion as we "paddle" and they look after me. Finally they took me home and decided to build me a greenhouse for my last days – and as we worked on it their concepts about such particular work became very active and could clearly be seen, and one of their conclusions was that "this will keep us going for when you are over the other side."

Q.   *This appears to be drama with an additional aim or purpose. Are you really identifying a form of assessment?*

Yes, we can see some of the diagnostic power of dramatic methods. It can readily be used to test what information people already possess, while assessing the next stages of instruction, and can be an excellent guide for diagnosis of the conceptual maturity, as well as to reveal social sensitivity. And of course it is not a tool for the mentally handicapped only. I can set things up – I cannot know the mentally handicapped in the same dimensions as the medical and caring staffs. To me those children and adults are "thous," as Martin Buber would express it in *I and Thou*[1], and must be treated as such or I lose honour for myself and them. I cannot use them as "its" or there can be no honour won in our acquaintance. To treat a person as a "thou" demands first that he be recognised fully as an individual with rights in the situation of our meeting. And rights means giving to people the power to affect a situation, to respond in a growing complexity of ways to that situation. One therefore has to be able to structure that situation in ways which enable this complexity to develop. I do not know how complex their powers of negotiation can become, because usually the real situation is not fully geared for this kind of progress to be undertaken. This is partly a result of too many people to be looked after at once, partly because the physical caring is stressed (and it needs to be), often though at the cost of the mental stretching. It possibly needs a whole new breed of staffing to be developed in our mental hospitals, the teacher-nurse. What a fascinating course that would be to develop!

I sympathise with those who find this kind of work too intrusive, too upsetting to the developed power patterns in hospital relationships which have come about because of the need these people have to be kept safe, looked after physically and controlled in the warmest sense for the good of all the residents. We have choices. We can decide to protect into ineffectiveness and keep people safe, and the place on an even keel, or we can systematically break this pattern at some cost to everyone. I am never sure whether "happy cabbages" are preferable to "emergent exploratory people." Nor have I the power to decide. I am an amateur among professionals. I can only say to myself when I ask that question of myself, "please life, let me participate in my living existence."

REFERENCES
1. *I and Thou*. Martin Buber. T. Clark, Edinburgh, 1970.
FILM: *Albert*, produced in conjunction with the National Association for the Mentally Handicapped.

5

Dramatherapy with Multi-handicap

SUE JENNINGS

Q. *You are a pioneer in dramatherapy. How do you define its role?*

At the beginning I must state my basic philosophy of the importance of drama for all, whether dysfunctioning or otherwise, and the contemporary social need for utilising all the resources at our disposal in some coherent way, including those of professional and amateur theatre, drama teachers and dramatherapists.

Many specialists in education and medicine, while accepting the importance of drama with many disadvantaged groups, have felt it to be inappropriate in the field of gross handicaps. However, having worked with an age range from pre-school to psycho-geriatric and with every type of handicap, mental illness and social disability, I have been convinced that there are:

"no physical or mental barriers to participating in drama."[1]

I propose to discuss the more specific area of dramatherapy application with multi-handicap, also realising that there is a wide range of disability often collected under this umbrella. I do not propose to discuss at length definitions of dramatherapy or to produce a catalogue of techniques. As far as definitions go I shall merely quote the definition of dramatherapy that has been accepted by the British Asociation of Dramatherapy:

Dramatherapy is a means of helping to understand and alleviate social and psychological problems, mental illness and handicap; and of facilitating symbolic expression through which man may get in touch with himself "both as individual and group" through creativity structures involving vocal and physical communication.

Dramatherapy skills include techniques of theatre, dance, mime, movement, psycho/socio-drama, role play, games, simulations, improvisation in both verbal and non-verbal expression.

Dramatherapy theory has developed from theories of creativity, drama, psychodynamics, analytic group psychotherapy, group dynamics, ritual, symbolism, the growth movement, and the new therapies.

Dramatherapists recognise the preventive value of drama in the community and school.

Dramatherapists believe that they must be both artist and therapist.

Within the wide range of therapeutic application of drama, and the many skills which can be drawn upon, there must always be the notion of creativity which is of course a part of recreation. When considering the multi-handicapped child, it is the creative process that we shall be considering rather than the psychotherapeutic one[2] as being more appropriate to the particular needs of this client group.

Q. *There must be many difficulties when introducing drama to people with serious handicap?*

When we are discussing leisure for any group in the community, what we are continually striving for is an enrichment of our lives; the interests we may have, the hobbies we may follow are of this category. Our advantage is that we have a choice — a very wide range of leisure choices both in terms of personal resources and community facilities.

When we are thinking in terms of work for the disabled, immediately personal choice and resources are more limited, and community facilities are often sadly lacking; too often leisure facilities are imposed on the individual rather like the proverbial dose of salts, because "it is good for you." Furthermore, the environment within which the handicapped are placed will often work against life enrichment and can on occasions cause additional problems.

Before we can think further, we have to understand the frustration and despair of parents and staff working in the long term with the severely handicapped. The physical demands are very time consuming, the frustrations of one way communication don't encourage the most enlightened of staff and the available resources in terms of training and provision are low down on the list of priorities.

In my experience from those who have attended training programmes and are working with the severely disabled, they are hungry for technique, support, new ideas and developments. At the moment, in terms of both training in this area and available literature, these are sparse.

Q.   *How do we get over to authorities the need for leisure occupation and its enjoyment?*

In Western society we still have a sharp divide between work and leisure; what falls into leisure categories is usually to be enjoyed and therefore less important than work that is not meant to be enjoyed but is more important. However, without a balance of the two, man is impoverished indeed. In fact we know that drama makes an important contribution to his whole development.[3]

We must also remember that learning can take place effectively if the process is enjoyable; so although we may be talking about the recreational aspects of drama it is necessary to be aware of the possible learning goals within that framework so that it can be utilised to the full.

It is difficult for us to get away from the reaction of having to justify something that is enjoyable. A colleague of mine was dismissed from a post as dramatherapist in an institution, by the consultant, because her clients laughed too much! It was pointed out to her that therapy was a serious business and the patients' levity was not appropriate.

Guilt at enjoyment perhaps could be considered under social values. An anthropological definition of socialisation is:

"The inculcation of the skills and attitudes necessary for playing given social roles."[4]

The socialisation process in any society will inextricably be bound up with the value system of that society — children's games, parental attitudes and models, education through schooling, television, literature — all of which play a part in the socialisation process. They differ from society to society because value systems vary throughout the world.

Unfortunately, in our society, there is an emphasis on dependency both in normal children and in the disabled of all ages. Therefore activities which encourage personal autonomy and independence are not on the list of priorities. Although the severely disabled will never be completely independent, I think it is our responsibility to encourage this as much as possible and the dramatherapeutic process is invaluable in developing its growth.

Two aspects of socialisation are:

1. Social skill learning — not only referring to motor skills but all types of skill we need to function in social situations; what could be called role-rehearsal for life; appropriate ways to behave in given situations;

2. Problem-solving — not just referring to an actual problem but problem-solving in the generic sense; if problems can be solved

through drama in many different ways, it facilitates the problem-solving capacity of the person.

Q.   *If we speak of social skills, this covers a whole range*
     of learning and participation which one senses is
     missing for the seriously disabled person.

This activity can be a part of the socialisation process and for the normal child happens often without forethought. Ingredients in schooling and in balanced home lives cater for the cultural experiences of the child, such as theatre, literature, music, art and so on, both to see and to participate in.

How often is it considered relevant for the severely disabled? Pop music is usually the norm, story reading is not frequent, and visual art in terms of the environment, especially in institutions, is rarely considered. When it is considered, how often is the client's personal choice taken into consideration? Again, autonomy is sadly lacking; a lot of culture that is available is imposed and frequently does not progress beyond pop culture.

I have frequently encountered extreme misery with the disabled adult who has had to contend with a "loss of culture"; one of my clients now in an institution with a passion for Beethoven has to mentally and emotionally switch off at non-stop Radio 1; another turns his face to the wall at the insistence of sport and comedy shows: his interests lie in documentaries and news features.

Let us remember to share to the full not only our own culture but that of others as a part of enriching the lives of the severely disabled.

Q.   *How do you apply the techniques of dramatherapy?*

The structure of any session is going to depend on an understanding of the particular client group and the goals of the session. None of this can happen in an arbitrary way and it is necessary to have a workable structure within which experimental drama can happen.

Although it will vary from group to group, normally a framework which has the right ingredients of stimulation and relaxation is appropriate. Chaotic sessions have resulted from the inexperienced practitioner concentrating on the stimulus, the "high" without giving sufficient balance to the "middle" and "low" areas. The most usual pattern that I use starts from relaxation, builds up to one or more climaxes and then has ample time for de-climax so that the group is peaceful at closing time. I have written elsewhere[5] on the idea that ritual and exploration are two ways of identifying the content of a session.

Ritual being the safe known area—the favourite game, the group dance, the special piece of music and so on—this serves as a safe boundary within which exploration can happen. Exploration is complementary to the ritual, it is discovery, there are risks, unknowns. A lot of our problem-solving drama comes into this area.[6]

Some of our clients have so ritualised a life that it has become no longer a shared experience but internalised, destructive and individual such as head banging, flicking and so on; or else the whole environment has become ritualised so that it is no longer a positive secure experience but has become institutionalised and results in depersonalisation and loss of affect. Frequently staff themselves fall into the institution trap and need to preserve their own security by keeping everything the same. Even physical movement of patients can become a threat to them.[7]

When ritual has reached this state it is no longer meaningful and therefore non-ritual.

Some of the Goals in Dramatherapy Application are:

1. to express and share feelings;
2. to stimulate the imagination;
3. to develop social skills;
4. to develop perception;
5. to allow decision making;
6. to encourage problem solving capacity;
7. to combat institutionalisation;
8. sheer enjoyment and pleasure;
9. to develop communication and relationships.

I would like to discuss just some of these goals more specifically in relation to:

(*a*) the multi-handicapped child who has severe intellectual damage.

Physical handling is very important for this group to provide a means of communication of love and trust which many severely handicapped children have never experienced. Building relationships through movement[8] is an important starting point in order to be able to proceed to more developed work *as a means of expressing and sharing feelings*—it is easy to forget when a child is severely damaged and may not be able to verbalise that he or she still has feelings to express. Very often with severe handicap there are also severe emotional problems—through reaction of parents, early hospitalisation or the effects of institutionalisation. However severe the disability, we must remember the strength of feelings; it is not that there are no feelings to communicate. Many will never acquire speech and non-verbal communication though movement, touch and sound can enable sorrow, rage, love, despair, all to be expressed *as a means of social skill learning* — however simple the skill, it can be rehearsed through the drama process to both reinforce the learning and make the experience enjoyable. The learning will be directed to specific skills so the structure will be comparatively "tight"; eating, dressing, teeth cleaning, can all be experienced through play and drama and then applied to the real life situation. Physical movement is important to develop control and balance; a sense of body image.[9] Various social situations to be encountered such as outings, holidays — all can be rehearsed through the drama in our rehearsal of life. *Developing relationships* — the actual drama process can facilitate relationships between all those concerned with the child; those who make up the child "social atom"; this of course will vary from child to child — for many their social atom is very minimal — especially if they have been abandoned and institutionalised; varieties of roles within the drama can enhance the roles a child encounters and relates to. I have found parents get tremendous satisfaction from being able to participate in drama with their child and utilising it as a means of expressing and sharing their feelings too.

(*b*) those with less severe/no intellectual impairment:

There are two major problems which manifest themselves in work with these groups:

Frustration — to have some understanding of one's problem but to feel helpless is a very daunting prospect; often the handicap is compounded by clients becoming depressed, irritable and violent.

Low self-image — especially in the field of human relationships; to know that one will never have a normal relationship and yet is capable of normal emotional responses both lead to low self image and often extreme rage.

If we can anticipate these responses in the young child we can start to use drama in a preventive way. It can be an important channel of expression too. Even the most violent of feelings can be worked through in drama as long as the session is carefully structured. Often there is relief at being just able to share these feelings and it does not have to be on a purely verbal level. Symbolic expression is a key concept to this work.

Self-esteem can be increased through satisfactory experiences in drama; the achievement of a totality; of something pleasurable; of combating the most rigorous of challenges (problem-solving again), and we have to remember that everything is possible through drama, through the imagination and the symbolic process.

To condense two important aspects of dramatherapy with these children — we can use dramatherapy as:

1 . A means of understanding emotional problems which may have been heightened by the handicap but not necessarily its cause; perhaps stemming from early rejection; or coming to terms with trauma after an accident.

2 . Helping them to adjust their perception of themselves and those around them and pave the way towards healthy relationships.

> Q. *Many of these children will be in institutions which have rules and customs. Is there not a danger that new insights create their own problems within the institutional set-up?*

We are all aware of the many processes that work against adequate development of the institutionalised child[10] and can see how the utilising of all the drama resources can help to combat this. However, until systems can change, we must not so disrupt an environment that in the end the child suffers. More of course is needed to educate the type of staff who work in institutions, but on the other hand it is futile to antagonise them. Frequently a compromise will be necessary, and those involved in drama will have to be expert at role-playing the diplomat and conciliator: it should be part of their skills!

One aspect, however, which I think needs a little more attention here is the type of behaviour often encountered in institutions with the multi-handicapped, and that is individual, compulsive ritual behaviour. Sometimes it is punished, other times it is sedated, or just ignored unless a child is causing itself actual physical harm.

I have found in many cases that the behaviour will decrease once a communication has been established — usually with one other — and the destructive movement can be shared and then turned into something more positive. Often it seems to be a task of finding a "way in" to the isolation and misery which can be preserved by complete withdrawal or else extreme violence, and developing trust and sharing. This can be a very painstaking and lengthy business, but one that can be fruitful if persevered. Very often a child will only "come out" on his own terms and this takes time. However, a way of starting I have discovered is to find what social distance the child will tolerate without moving away, and then to mirror the same movement as the child; often one will be allowed to move nearer and hopefully eye contact will then take place. Then one can start to vary the movement (or sound) and it will become less obsessional and compulsive and begin to be built on shared experience.

As John Blacking said, "Aren't music and dance important in themselves? Isn't culture a product of sharing, not of individuality? Therefore can't we look at movement and dance as a formal expression of order which is the basis of humanity?"[11]

Q.   *How do you see the future for this shared experience?*

The future? Obviously one would like to predict that attitudes will change; certainly attitudes seem to be changing towards both the handicapped and dramatherapy[12] but it is not easy to predict whether there will be more resources.

However, great strides could be made at least by the various specialists concerned with the lives and well-being of the severely disabled being able to communicate together for the common concern of their client. The Dartington seminar has already demonstrated that there is a common goal, which is very encouraging.

Specifically in the field of applying dramatherapy we need the joint resources of the actor, both professional and amateur, the drama teacher and the dramatherapists, as all have an important function in the lives of the severely disabled.

I am not being partisan when I refer specifically to drama — it happens to be my particular skill. I frequently work in conjunction with art therapists, music therapists and a variety of disciplines in the caring and teaching professions.

However, it is time for the drama people to communicate with each other and work for the common good, especially for the multi-handicapped child who is so low on the list of priorities in contemporary society.

Already the music, art and drama therapists are sitting round a table discussing areas of common concern and realising that their skills are complementary rather than competitive.

Let us hope that the future will bring about greater communication between all those concerned with the well-being of children, but especially those concerned with enriching the life of the child who has multiple handicaps.

> "If a man does not keep pace with his companions,
> perhaps it is because he hears a different drummer.
> Let him step to the music he hears,
> however measured or far away."
> — THOREAU

46   *The Arts and Disabilities*

REFERENCES

1. Jennings, S. 1973 (i). *Remedial Drama* (Pitman's).
2. Jennings, S. 1978 (ii). "Dramatherapy: The Anomalous Profession" in *The Journal of Dramatherapy*, Vol. 1, No. 4.
3. Courtney, R. 1974. *Play, Drama and Thought* (Cassels).
4. Mayer, P. 1970. "Socialisation and the Social Anthropologist" in ASA Monograph No. 8.
5. Jennings, S. 1973 (iii). "Ritual and Exploration" in *Times Educational Supplement*, 7.12.73.
6. Jennings, S. 1973 (ii). "Ritual and its Links with Performance" (Dramatherapy Conference 1973).
7. Jennings, S. 1975. "The Importance of the Body in Non-Verbal Methods of Therapy" in *Creative Therapy*, ed. Jennings (Pitman's).
8. Sherborne, V. 1975. "Building Relationships through Movement," *ibid.*
9. Jennings, S. 1973 (iv). "The Special Nursery: Explorations in Creative Play for Young Severely Handicapped Children" in *Drama in Education: 2*, ed. Hodgson and Banham (Pitman's).
10. Wright, J. 1978. "A case for Drama with Institutionalised Sub-Normal Children" in *Journal of Dramatherapy*, Vol. 1, No. 3.
11. Blacking, J. 1974. "Music, Dance and the Growth of Man," RCA Lecture.
12. Jennings, S. 1978 (i). "Dramatherapy with the Physically Handicapped" in *Drama in Therapy*, ed. Courtney and Schattner (in press, Drama Book Specialists, NY).

The Journal of Dramatherapy is published by the British Association of Dramatherapy and is available from 7 Hatfield Road, St Albans, Herts.

6

Drama with the Blind Adult

DAVID MUMFORD

Q. *To start a course using drama with blind students requires determination and imagination on the part of everyone concerned. What is the philosophy and aim behind such a dramatic venture?*

In order to appreciate fully the philosophy behind drama with the blind, it is important to have some basic knowledge of blindness, and the unique functional problems it imposes on the individual. To be labelled "blind" does not, as is frequently assumed, mean to be totally without sight; the statutory definition as set out in the 1948 Act[1] is "to be unable to perform work for which eyesight is essential," which basically means that some blind people can see, or are referred to as having useful residual vision. This is particularly applicable to a high proportion of those over retirement age, for blindness and advancing years are synonymous. The same, however, cannot be said for braille and blindness since only ten per cent of all those registered as blind possess the necessary aptitude to read braille. This kind of "textbook" information is useful, but what is of paramount importance to the consumer is the attitude and approach of the dispenser, and here lies the major key to the success of drama with the blind.

It all began in 1974 when, during the academic holidays, I was invited to run an activities project for visually handicapped school children. Integration is a major problem for the visually handicapped and so it was felt attempts should be made to integrate blind and sighted children from the same area of Wolverhampton, using drama as the vehicle. Practical sessions were held at a local Day Centre for the Blind and created a great deal of interest amongst the adult blind attending the centre. Their comments and my own assessment of the scheme motivated me to organise the first residential drama school for the blind.

During August 1975, eighteen registered blind people travelled from all over the country to Coventry's Belgrade Studio Theatre to participate in the school, the aim of which was to give the widest possible concept of theatre in the time available. Apart from an extension of theatre techniques, students demonstrated how physical as well as social confidence can be developed, together with a sense of achievement and realisation of their own potential and capabilities.

Surprisingly, some of the most popular sessions were those dealing with movement and dance, when formal mobility aids were abandoned and the pleasures of unrestricted, yet disciplined movement experienced, generating confidence and a great sense of release. The newly blind are naturally cautious in their movement and such sessions allow the full vocabulary of movement to be explored and the pleasures in rhythm and dance re-established; and for the congenitally blind, movement sessions can help to give a basic alphabet of movements previously denied them by their inability to absorb body language visually, to personalise and reproduce it.

The course tutors were personal friends, professionally connected with either the theatre or drama, but none having had previous experience of working with visually handicapped people. From an initial group of nine, emerged a small core who possessed the right qualities and attitudes to work with the visually handicapped and these have remained with me as tutors on both summer schools and subsequent weekend projects. Students expressed great enthusiasm for the initial and later summer schools, giving opinions and comments through questionnaires and personal letters. Their suggestions reinforced certain priorities which were beginning to emerge in the minds of the tutors; mainly that this type of work should be spread over as many areas of the country as possible and with the emphasis on increasing the individual's movement and mobility skills.

Locally based weekend courses were devised, and seen as a way of spreading the benefit to as many blind people as possible. Such courses, though, would need to have a slightly different emphasis than the summer schools, since a high proportion of students attending would be both the elderly and newly blind.

Q.   *What then are the main aims of the weekend project?*

The first is to establish personal confidence, then to increase body awareness and orientation skills—leading to increased mobility. It is important then to confirm the need for continued use of gesture and facial expression, to develop a greater awareness to vocal subtleties, and to provide a creative outlet for possible suppressed frustrations and desires. Finally, we seek to provide the stimulus for a regular group for added social interaction.

Q. *How do you put your aims into practice?*

On each of the weekend courses, a group of twenty students are sub-divided and receive instruction relating to voice/body on a turnabout system. We explore individual and group physical potentials through : limber/body awareness exercises; improvised movement to music and exploration of simple dance through rhythmic patterns. The potentials of voice are explored through: correct breathing; developing an awareness to resonance/articulation/modulation and improvised speech. Whilst it may appear that these are compartmentalised, attempts are made to overlap and show positive connections between both vocal and physical powers of communication. It is interesting to note that few blind people, particularly the congenitally blind, are aware of the need for and value of non-verbal communication. In fact, a large proportion of this latter group seem totally unaware that the body, in addition to the voice, is a communicating tool. And it is therefore on this premise that the movement sessions of our courses are based. The first day of any course must include fun exercises and games to aid positive group interaction and build individual confidence by breaking through those inevitable inhibiting barriers of shyness. Once a relaxed and conducive atmosphere develops amongst the group, personalities not only become more natural, but true creativity then materialises. Towards the end of our workshops tutors are able to encourage the interpretation of music through movement, possibly linked with extensive speech improvisation and creative dance dramas.

One must not forget that tension is often present in human beings, especially when physical activity is taking place. With the visually handicapped, natural tensions are accentuated and therefore significant emphasis is placed on acquiring relaxation skills to be used both during the weekend workshops or the summer school, but more importantly on an individual basis at home.

An exciting new dimension to our weekend workshops is an experimental attempt at linking the sense of touch with imaginative creativity. Vacuum formed shapes of handling size with undulating surfaces are given to students for exploration. One shape in particular had concave and convex areas upon which had been added not only contrasting textures but also vivid colours. Using the sense of touch and her remaining vision, a student was inspired to describe a remarkable

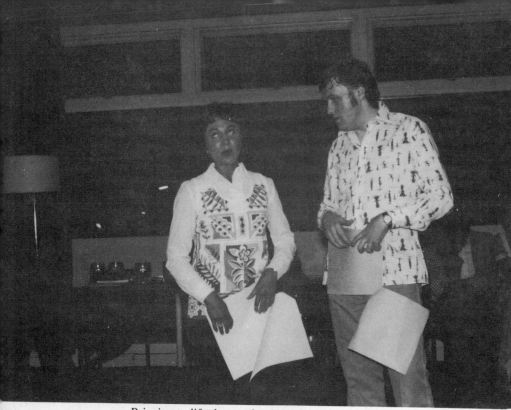

Bringing to life the words of another using braille scripts

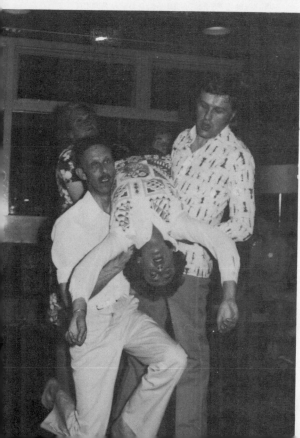

Conclusion to
a creative dance drama

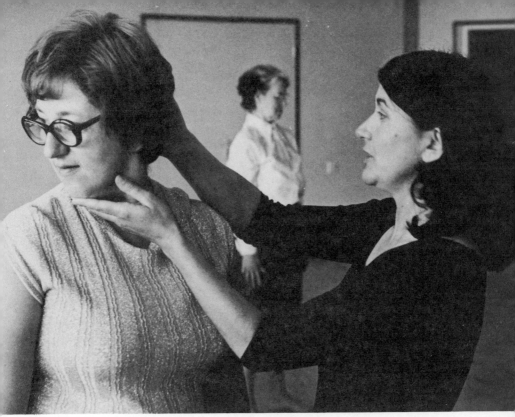

Positive feedback is given to students during posture and body awareness exercises

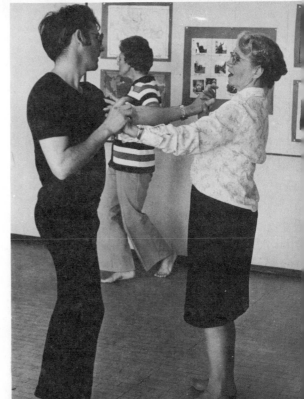

For the elderly blind
the pleasures in natural
rhythm need encouragement

Photos by Middlesex County Press

location of hills and valleys, covered in a variety of shrubbery. An emotional reaction to the clearly imagined scene was added and displayed total involvement with the shape. The whole group then participated in exploring "the imaginary location" and coupled their own individual response to it. A group discussion ensued and resulted in an exciting improvisation.

The visually handicapped students attend an initial series of three concentrated weekend workshops, but the success of an ongoing group is dependent upon the collaboration of two specialists: one, a specialist worker with the blind, possibly the mobility officer, whose awareness and knowledge of the problems relating to movement and mobility of the visually handicapped is important, and the second, a drama specialist.

Together, as a team, they are introduced to our methods and principles of work through observing and participating in the first weekend workshop; collaborating with us during the second, then finally conducting their own sessions under our guidance and support. Following these introductory weekends the leaders are then able to forge ahead with a regular group, developing and expanding our basic philosophies of drama with the blind.

> Q. *The specialists will presumably need some intro-*
> *duction or training for the work, and this could*
> *create problems as it grows. How will you deal with*
> *this development?*

An Advisory Group[2] has been formed to encourage the development of the work and is arranging a residential course for drama specialists interested in working with the visually handicapped. The course will involve an assessment of the candidate's abilities to engage successfully in drama; with training concentrating on the practical implications a visual handicap imposes on both the individual and the group, and candidates will have the opportunity of working directly with a group of blind people. Prior to the course candidates will be encouraged to develop the necessary close liaison with the specialist worker with the visually handicapped in their area.

Identifiable labels seem to be important in today's society and certainly this is true where innovatory work is concerned. We have long sought a suitable label, not only to define our work to various authorities, but more importantly to the consumer. We feel that we fit snugly between educational and recreational: educational — meaning the development of one or all of a person's powers of mind and body; and recreational — meaning to reinvigorate the mind and body. We discourage the linking of the word therapeutic to our work since this implies the curative and preventative treatment of disease; this does not accord with the ethos towards which we aspire. Blindness is a consequence of disease or accident and is usually an irreversible condition to which the individual needs to adapt. However, involvement with drama for anyone, whether handicapped, disadvantaged or otherwise, can be therapeutic, but our emphasis is towards the functional problems of the visually handicapped, for it is these that separate and influence society's attitudes and responses to blind people.

Q. *How do you view the results of the courses?*

Perhaps the responses of the visually handicapped themselves can best sum up the impact they have experienced from participating in drama with the blind:

"It was a joy to move with such freedom — no, with such abandonment — again. To hear my voice filling the four corners of a room again instead of barely raised above a whisper, to lift my head up and move, if not with grace and elegance, at least with certainty and assurance."

"Movement and Mime — this was for me the most exciting part of the course . . . there was something so indescribably releasing and absorbing, relaxing and exhilarating beyond everyday experience, that it was worth every ounce of aching muscle."

REFERENCES
1. *The National Assistance Act 1948*, Part 3, Section 29. HMSO.
2. Advisory Group for Drama with the Blind, linked with the Royal National Institute for the Blind, London.

   Qualified drama tutors interested in such work can gain details from the Advisory Group, c/o Mr C. J. Attrill, Sports & Recreation Officer, Royal National Institute for the Blind, 224-8 Great Portland Street, London W1N 6AA.

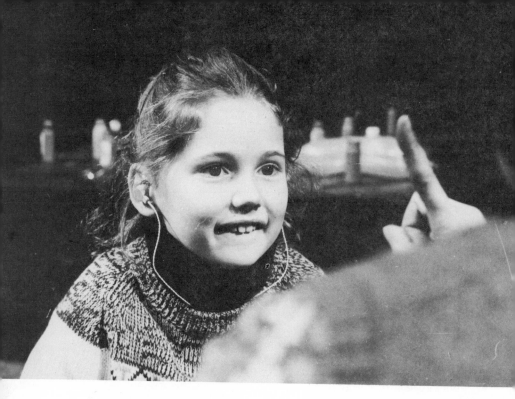

Working with deaf children in the Scottish Festival of Mime

Photos by Scotsman Publications Ltd

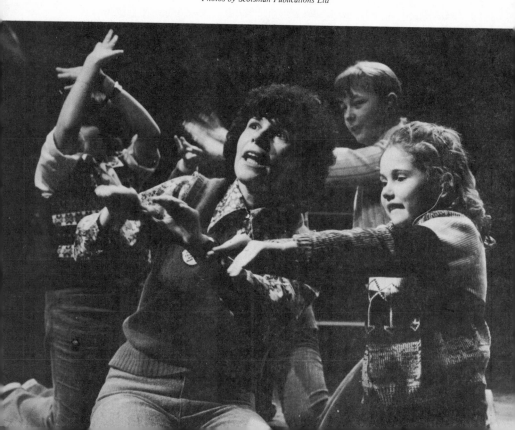

7

Mime with the Deaf

PAT KEYSELL

Q. *The teaching of the deaf is a very crucial task not made easier by the differing views and approaches of the oral and manual schools of thought. What are your reactions in working with deaf people?*

I always speak or write about working with deaf people with very mixed feelings nowadays, because I am so aware of how much they prefer to speak for themselves. The leaders who emerged from the British Theatre of the Deaf, particularly those who have taken the ADB Special Training Course (Associate of the Drama Board) are now organising and running their own projects, and this is how it should be. The whole emphasis and development in the education of the deaf has been towards independence and integration, and the theatre is an important area where this can happen, although there are still many problems.

Another important qualification is concerned with the danger of making generalised statements. There are so many different degrees of deafness, ranging from partial hearing loss to those who were born deaf, or were deafened in infancy. Add to this the great range of personality and character which can influence reaction to deafness — not to mention personal endowment — and it becomes quite useless to talk about "working with the deaf" as if it were just one category. It is fairly true to say, however, that most of the children and adults I have worked with have come within the "severely deaf" or "deaf to all speech" category, and so the points I have to make are influenced by that fact.

It may be helpful to begin by summarising some of the most common problems caused by severe deafness from an early age:

1. Language deprivation. Deaf children cannot "pick up" words naturally as hearing children do.

2. Lack of mental stimulation which hearing people get from sound — approach of a car, or clatter of tea cups; above all, music.

3. Frustration at not being understood, or not being able to understand what is being said, with consequent aggression.

4. Isolation.

5. Receptivity and dependence.

On the other hand, there are positive compensations, such as:

1. Acute powers of observation, plus a very retentive memory for visual information.

2. Good physical co-ordination. Deafness can cause a certain heaviness or clumsiness, but this can be dealt with. I have certainly found that deaf people learn mime technique much more quickly than the hearing do.

3. Great expressive power with body, face and hands.

4. A sense of humour (which can be cruel) but is also connected with an overdeveloped sense of the absurd. One has only to watch a conductor and a full-sized orchestra on TV with the sound turned off to realise how this comes about.

5. An intense inner life which is not dissipated by constant chatter.

> Q. *You are a skilled mime artiste. Why is mime valuable to a deaf child in particular?*

If we look at a definition of mime (this is not my definition but it is my favourite one):

> "The 'outer' world contains objects, people, animals, organic life of all sorts, the sum and substance of our environment. The 'inner' world consists of our feelings, thoughts, impulses, dreams. The art of Mime begins where and when these two worlds meet."[1]

then it becomes obvious that deaf people are the best possible candidates for the art of mime; that here is something they can not only do to a standard of excellence, but be seen to be doing it.

In developing my method of teaching mime to deaf children, I was endeavouring to overcome their disadvantages and make the most of the positive compensations.[2] For instance, there are some children whose language deprivation is so severe that they cannot even answer a simple question such as "What is your name?" All they can do is repeat the question, or try to, because imitation and repetition is all that they think is required of them. But these same children, if confronted by a similar situation in terms of action – what is the next step? how can this problem be solved? – can make the required leap and come up with an answer.

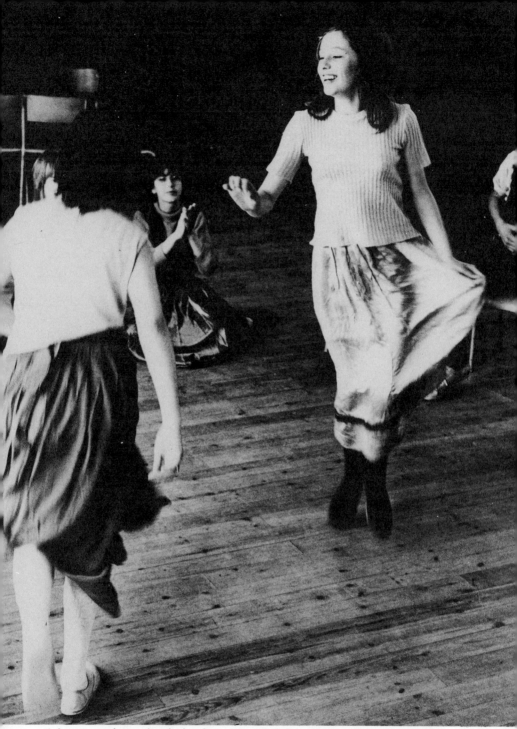

A happy respite as the gipsies dance around their camp fire: from a mime play about gipsies improvised by severely deaf children in the Newham School for the Deaf

Photo by Rob Inglis

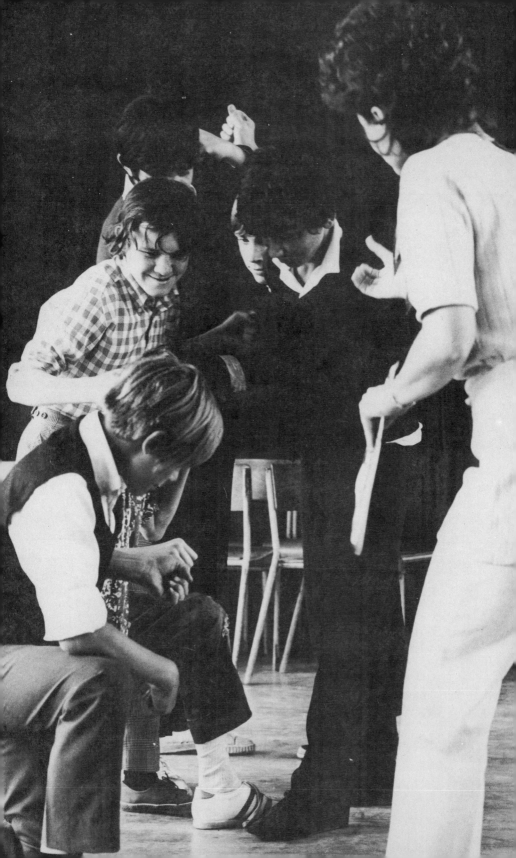

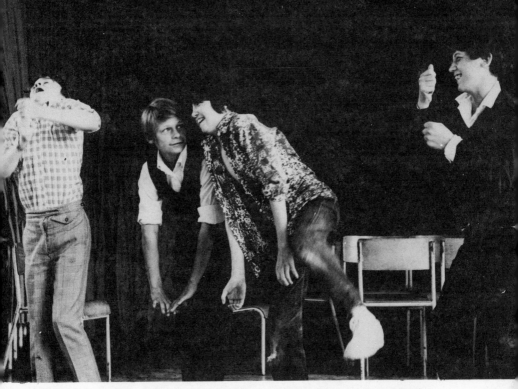

A mime improvised by the boys in Newham School for the Deaf was based on the training of American marines culminating in the invasion of Okinawa. The two pictures show (*left*) the assault course, and (*above*) the planting of the American flag on the island

Photos by Rob Inglis

I evolved a series of very simple mime games to get over the idea that everyone has to make their own contribution, not merely imitate me or each other. These worked very well, and in time I was amazed to see how original and inventive the children could be. I am sure that this work, executed in mime, gave them a mental stimulus and sense of sequence and structure which can be very helpful in the understanding of language, and the way language is used in communication.

Mime can also offer relief from the great strain of trying to lip-read. Lip-reading is a gift; not all children have it. But in mime, we perceive and understand because of what we see happening. Everyone is included. Instead of frustration, aggression, isolation, we have an outpouring of expression — spontaneity — co-operation, and freedom from dependence.

Expression through mime can help the children to come to terms with their experience. They know far more than they can ever express in words. This can be put into action. It helps to develop flexibility of mind; a shape, or a line, quickly drawn on the blackboard can be interpreted in many different ways. A story can be recreated with a different ending. This helps to counteract the rigid, literal approach which can result from the formal and artificial learning of language; the tendency to seize on one meaning for each word, overlooking the subtlety and variation that language can encompass, particularly in different contexts and where speech is concerned, with intonation. Intonation is replaced by quality of movement.

We should also not underestimate the importance for everyone to succeed at something; non-academic children can excel at something creative like mime; they know when they do something well and this gives them enormous pleasure, with the added bonus of giving pleasure to others.

Q.   *Problems must accentuate in adulthood. How can theatre help to alleviate the frustrations?*

The problems caused by deafness can become even more acute as the child grows up. Although many adults may appear to have achieved remarkably balanced lives, with a well paid job, running a home, family, a car — behind the facade there is still enormous deprivation. "Man cannot live by bread alone." The lack of cultural background is very obvious; the suffering caused by public attitudes is not so obvious. I know that many young deaf people feel tremendously let down when they come to realise that the integration, held out like a tantalizing carrot throughout their school days, will never come to pass.

However, some of the talented deaf performers in the British Theatre of the Deaf (and now in the Interim Theatre Company) have proved that a high standard of creative work can break through these barriers. On stage there is a lively mind at work, an engaging personality, a great warmth and humour comes across; after the show, members of the audience want to meet the actors, there is much to talk about and problems of communication are forgotten.

As well as pure mime, movement and dance, the company uses a medium called sign-mime, based on the natural sign language of the deaf. Although limited in vocabulary, the sign language is rich in mimetic gesture and expressive power; the limited vocabulary can be extended by mime, and the lack of grammatic structure becomes irrelevant when interpreting poetry or poetic dialogue. Deaf people are very proud of their sign language, and they love to teach it to the hearing. We found that we all gained great insight into the meaning of language by striving to find the best possible physical expression for a particular concept behind a word, or phrase, in context. I personally believe that it is possible to reach a profound level of communication through this use of sign language.

Q. *Even with this breakthrough the difficulties must be
as tremendous as the progress.*

Many problems remain. A deaf theatre company will always attract
numbers of deaf people in the audience; the cultural and educational
impoverishment of that audience makes it extremely difficult, if not
impossible, to present material which will also attract and satisfy a
hearing audience. To perform only for deaf people would be to abandon
the long held ideal of integration; to perform only for the hearing would
amount to desertion of that section of the community who perhaps need
it most.

It was our policy in the Theatre of the Deaf for the deaf members to
take over as much of the organisation, business management and
administration of the company's work as possible, and here public
attitudes are not always so accommodating. I have known occasions
when managers and publicity representatives have objected to the
incidence of having to deal with a deaf person. In this day and age it
seems unforgiveable, but we have to bear in mind that there is still a
deep-seated fear of the handicap in people who have had no previous
contact with it. There is still a great deal to be done in educating the
public and bringing about more contact so that this fear is removed.

But it cannot be just one-sided. The behaviour of handicapped people
is sometimes difficult to accept, even by those most inclined towards
them. As far as deaf people are concerned, the ordinary human faults
and frailties can become intensified to quite a strong degree; aggressive
attitudes, outbursts of temper and anger, rigid opinion, defence
mechanism, arrogance, plus the headlong approach, scathing frankness,
exaggerated facial expression and loud, unmodulated voices, can all be
very difficult to cope with. And very tiring. So where does it begin? Who
makes the most allowances? If more hearing people are prepared to try
to understand what it is like to be deaf, then perhaps more deaf people
will try to understand what it is like to be hearing.

As I mentioned at the beginning, some of the Drama Board Associates
are now running their own projects and making great headway. They are
the ambassadors. They are still learning, but at least the vicious circle has
been broken.

REFERENCES
1. *The Mime Book*. Claude Kipnis (1974). Harper Colophon Books.
2. *Motives for Mime*. Pat Keysell (1975). Evans.

NOTE:
A copy of a sixty minute video cassette on the development and work of the Theatre of the
Deaf is available on loan from the Carnegie Trust Office.

8

Music in Disability

ALASTAIR D. PYE

Q. *As an introduction to your talk at the seminar you had the 'experts' enjoying your class-work and participating easily, even if with a slight embarrassment. What is your approach to a typical lesson?*

There are varying disabilities in Special Schools and in hospitals and it has been found that residents have benefited generally from music therapy and general musical experiences. Here in the Central Region of Scotland many educationally sub-normal, severely sub-normal, partial-hearing and maladjusted pupils have enjoyed singing, singing-games, dancing and making music with tuned and untuned percussion instruments; they have enjoyed listening to the music they created on tape. Staff and students in the units also enjoy the musical experiences, for music brings different groups of pupils and staff together for a short time during the day — a time of enjoyment and relaxation. Songs can help overcome some rhythm problems (particularly with deaf and partial-hearing pupils) and help co-ordination and general awareness of environment.

When introducing music to educationally sub-normal, severely sub-normal, autistic and partial-hearing pupils, a bright, good-sized, well-ventilated room is preferable. A good piano is valuable as pupils can have a functional focal-point in the room which makes a clear, pleasant sound — something which will help them with singing as well as providing a positive background for games, action songs and dancing. Seats are best in a semicircle; everybody can see the pianist or singer and all have freedom for "stand-up or sit-down" movement. My lessons often begin by singing "Good Morning/Good Afternoon Everybody" to the descending form of the major scale (D' T L S F M R D). After this our approach to music will be through rhythm — basic hand-clapping. For this we can use "I'd like to teach the World to sing." We become more aware of our bodies by tapping knees, toes, heads or tickling the knees of the person next to us. The same or another 4/4 tune can be used. Pupils may laugh at the actions but this is good as it helps breathing and any subsequent singing will benefit. Perhaps it's now time for a simple Action Game, one where parts of the body are used, such as:

Heads, Shoulders, Knees and Toes —
Raise your Hands above your Head.
If you're happy and you know it
Clap your Hands.

Pupils and residents will now be ready for a short rest so the piano can play a restful song, "Sing a Rainbow," while heads are lowered as if sleeping. Staff can sing the words of the song. Our session is nearly finished so it can be rounded off by singing "Good Morning Everybody" as sung at the beginning of the session. If the pupils have now to leave the room they can march out to one of Sousa's famous marches *Liberty Bell.*

Q. *With a range of disabilities in the children what are the difficulties?*

The partial hearing and deaf pupils present more of a problem for involvement with music, but once a successful means of presenting music has been found the benefits are considerable. The best approach to sessions is through rhythm. Clapping hands, tapping feet in time to music is a good way to begin. Once again a good, clear piano is preferable. The pitch of keyboard material should be determined studying each pupil's audiogram. It has been found that one octave either side of middle C on the piano is suitable for most pupils. Simple melodies can be written on the board or overhead projector and they can be tapped while the rhythm names are said aloud. This contributes considerably to speech improvement. The session material can be similar to that of the educationally sub-normal and severely sub-normal in choice of songs, singing games and movement. It is a good idea to take a specific project each month and choose material around it. Subjects should be selected where there may already be a basic vocabulary — for example:

Parts of the body   Pets
Food   Transport

Projects in art and crafts can be an added aid to follow up musical projects. Games such as "Musical Bumps" are fun — the pupils march round the room to music and when the music stops the last person on the floor is out. This contributes to general musical perception and the listening carefully to vibration from the piano or record player.

Many teachers cannot play piano or guitar or even sing but want to use music with disability. In this case they could contact a pianist or singer, get together to plan sessions which can then be taped, so producing accompaniment whenever it is required. If no instrumentalist or singer can be found, the local authority Music Adviser should be able to put a teacher in touch with the appropriate musicians. Music has a tremendous contribution to make in disability—pleasure, improved co-ordination and general awareness of environment. The more music the better!

NOTE:

The Music Adviser, Miss D. Kennard, at the Disabled Living Foundation (346 Kensington High Street, London W14 8NS: 01-602 2491) has a series of leaflets including:
  Music books related to handicapped people
  Working in music and training available
  Music for one-handed pianists
  Magazines and journals
  Publishers and publications
  Old Time Records and Song Music
  Musical Instruments
  Contacts, Libraries, Jobs and organisations.

LIST OF PUBLICATIONS AVAILABLE FOR MUSIC WITH CHILDREN

SONGS FOR CHILDREN

The Oxford Nursery Song Book. P. Buck. O.U.P.
The Oxford School Music Books. Books 1-3. R. Fiske *and* J. Dobbs. O.U.P.
Sing Together. W. Appleby *and* F. Fowler. O.U.P.
Children's Play Songs. P. Nordoff *and* C. Robbins. Theodore Presser Co. Pa.
Faith, Folk and Clarity. P. Smith. Galliard.
Folk Songs for Fun. O. Brand. Essex Music.

RECORDS WHICH MAY BE AVAILABLE

Bang on a Drum. BBC Playschool record. BBC Roundabout 17.
Children's Singing Games. Wilson and Gallacher. Topic Records IMP A 101.
Growing Up with Wally Whyton. Pye GGL 0285.
Singing Games and Party Songs for Children. John Longstaff. EMI 7EJ 266.
Songs for Singing Children. John Longstaff. EMI XLP 50008.
Songs for Children. Rowland and others. Argo DA 32.

HELP FOR TEACHERS

Children Make Music. R. Addison. Holmes McDougall.
Children's Traditional Singing Games. Books 1-5. Gomme & Sharp. Novello.
Ears and Eyes. Books 1-2. J. Dobbs, R. Fiske *and* M. Lane. O.U.P.

Exploring Sound — Creative Musical Projects for Teachers. J. Tillman. Stainer & Bell.
Our Friends the Animals. E Hughes. Novello.
Oxford School Music Books. Teachers' Manual. R. Fiske *and* J. Dobbs. O.U.P.
Ready to Play — Stories with percussion. J. Blades & C. Ward. BBC Publications.
Rhymes with Chimes. O. Rees *and* A. Mendoza. O.U.P.
Ring a Ding — Songs with tuned percussion. Y. Adair. Novello.
Singing Games for Recreation. Books 1-4. J. E. Tobbitt. A. & C. Black.
Things that Help Us. E. Hughes. Novello.

BOOKS ABOUT MUSIC FOR SLOW-LEARNING CHILDREN

Music therapy. J. Alvin. Hutchinson 1974.
Music for the handicapped child. J. Alvin. O.U.P. 1978.
Music Therapy for the Autistic Child. J. Alvin. O.U.P. 1978.
They can make music. P. Bailey. O.U.P. 1973.
Making musical instruments. K. M. Blocksidge. The Nursery Schools Assn. (89 Stamford Street, SE1.)
Voices and Instruments. Avril Dankworth. Hart Davis Educational 1973.
The slow learner and music. J. P. B. Dobbs. O.U.P. 1974.
Music, movement and mime for children. V. Gray *and* R. Percival. O.U.P. 1962.
Listen — Let's Make Music. Ann Hunt. Bedford Square Press 1976.
Music to help disabled children to move. D. Kennard *and* M. Gilbertson. A.P.C.P. Publications, 25 Goff's Park Road, Southgate, Crawley RH11 8AX. 1977.
Therapy in music for handicapped children. P. Nordoff *and* C. Robbins. Gollancz 1973.
Music therapy in action. M. Priestly. Constable 1974.
Musical instruments Made to be Played. R. Roberts. Dryad Press 1968.
Singing in Special Schools. D. Ward. Bedford Square Press 1973.
Hearts and Hands and Voices. D. Ward. O.U.P. 1976.
Songs of Speech. M. Warren *and* D. Spinks. Taskmaster Ltd., Morris Road, Leicester. 1977.

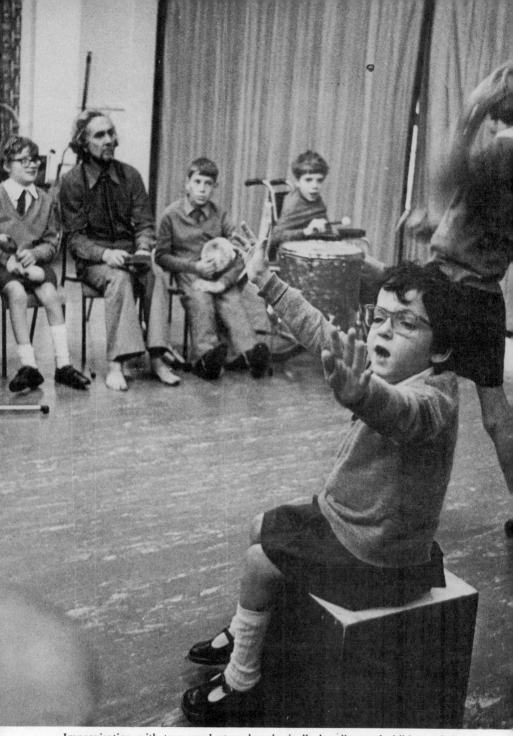

Improvisation with two conductors by physically handicapped children of the
Dame Hannah Rogers School, Ivybridge

Photo by Chris Schwarz

9

Music with the Handicapped

DAVID WARD

Q. *You have a wealth of experience in your specialisms of music and the training of children who are backward educationally. What are your overall impressions of the work?*

I think that in the field of care and education of the disabled there has been great progress in the last fifteen years. However, I would like to concentrate our thinking on looking forward, rather than on too much analysis of what we have tried to do already. To teach severely handicapped children, for example, is now a very respectable profession. These children are now considered to be educable, and education for them is at last intelligently organised and applied.

During 1978 there was a Special Schools Music Festival held at Dartington in the banqueting-hall. To this festival came 150 educationally subnormal children — both "mild" and "severe" — and for the best part of a day there was singing, dancing and the playing of instruments. Most of the small number of observers who attended this event remarked on the high standard of behaviour, the continuous attentiveness, and the clear enjoyment of these children.

Ten years ago, we might have been thought to be slightly irresponsible to attempt to bring mentally handicapped children into this beautiful hall for more than a few minutes, let alone to encourage them to sing and play there with energy. For a long time we have underestimated the abilities of these children in particular; indeed, I think it is true to say that we have underestimated the potential of most handicapped individuals.

One of the most important findings of the *Music for Slow Learners*[1] project was that the musical abilities of these children had been very much underestimated. Many examples of interesting music-making were recorded during the course of the project; these recordings show quite clearly that, in certain circumstances, slow learning children can achieve musical results which compare favourably with their normal peers.

These examples of good performance are, unfortunately, exceptional. Only in about 10% of the special schools surveyed were the children being suitably extended musically. The main reason for this seemed to be quite simply a lack of good teaching, and this is not so much the fault of the teaching profession but rather an administrative matter.

Examples of interesting work were found in schools where there was an expert musician, but also examples of high quality were found in schools in which the music teacher was not a "specialist" — indeed, some of these teachers had only moderate skills. Equipment, working spaces and resources did not appear to greatly affect the quality of the music activities in the schools; the teacher was the important factor, with the head teacher's active interest and support coming a close second.

Almost all the highly committed teachers complained that they were working in isolation and had no idea what they really could expect from their pupils or how their standards compared with those of similar groups. Interestingly, these teachers believed that their activities were not primarily aimed at making the children more musically proficient. The more important stated aims were to facilitate communication, to improve co-ordination, to foster socialisation, to give the children a greater sense of confidence, to improve their aural sense generally.

Q.   *What happens after school and is there a need for a link between school and community groups?*

The *Music for Slow Learners* project was essentially concerned with children of school age. It was, however, from the outset a great concern of many teachers and parents that provision for musical opportunities stopped short when the children left school. This was especially noticeable in the case of severely subnormal and physically handicapped children. For this reason, we felt that organisations such as Gateway Clubs and the Physically Handicapped and Able Bodied Clubs had an extra special need for musical activity. In the event, it was possible to offer music and arts tuition each year (1969-78) to the Devon PHAB course which has been held very successfully in Torbay and at Dartington Hall. I would like to focus attention today on this particular venture because I think it shows clearly where important needs lie, and perhaps points a way to meet some of these needs.

In the early PHAB courses, music was a very popular activity with the participants; more of them opted to do music than could be easily coped with. The activities consisted largely of the preparation of popular and folk songs with guitar and other instrumental backing, the learning of a simple instrument (e.g. the mouth-organ)—so that they would have something to take away with them, and the addition of music to plays, puppetry and films. More recently, the PHAB participants have tended to opt for art and craft—possibly a reflection of the expert tuition we were able to provide.

A video-film was made by a small group of physically handicapped participants of the PHAB course in 1975. At this course, only a few opted for music and these few were among the least able members of the course. We decided to make a simple film which would involve the addition of background music; the more this idea was discussed, the more they seemed to want to make a "documentary" film about themselves. In the event, we decided to film various aspects of the course itself and to bring in musical background where possible—e.g. to accompany a river trip, the arts activities and particularly a shadow puppet play.

I think the project showed clearly the need for children of this age group to firmly relate their music to other activities. There is a difficult problem in that, whilst the techniques they are able to cope with remain at a child level, the content must be much more "grown-up." A film project of this type affords just this opportunity.

Q. *You and your colleagues have a keen interest in bringing the various arts together in a form of teaching. How does this work?*

Integrating the arts is often a vague notion. It is, of course, important to try to do just this where handicapped participants are concerned because they need as many sensory inputs as possible. Integration of disciplines is more likely to succeed if the approach is based on the participants' needs rather than on a vague aesthetic ideal. It is possible that certain combinations of arts activities work naturally together, whilst others do not.

The new Carnegie project here at Dartington aims to explore ways in which this coming together can happen. The aims of the new project may be summarised as follows:

1 . To explore how the arts can contribute to the education and enrichment of life of handicapped children and young people. Particular emphasis will be laid on multi-sensory work which will evolve through a group of three teachers, practising the different arts and working together in consultation with each other and on common projects.

2 . To observe work in the same field being done elsewhere in Great Britain.

3 . To share experience with others through discussion and the organisation of short courses and conferences.

4 . To compile a report, illustrated by tapes, films and photographs, which will bring together the experience gathered.

5 . To collect together relevant resources of various kinds which will be available to all workers in the same field of education.

6 . To initiate on-going pieces of work, both teaching and research, in the College and other Centres.

As with the Music for Slow Learners, the new project will set out to be of service to those who teach, contributing not only to the world of the special school but to those who, in the normal education system, come across a wide variety of handicap and disadvantage.

Making marks means making moves: an example of the experimental work at the Dame Hannah Rogers School for Cerebral Palsied Children

Photo by Bruce Kent

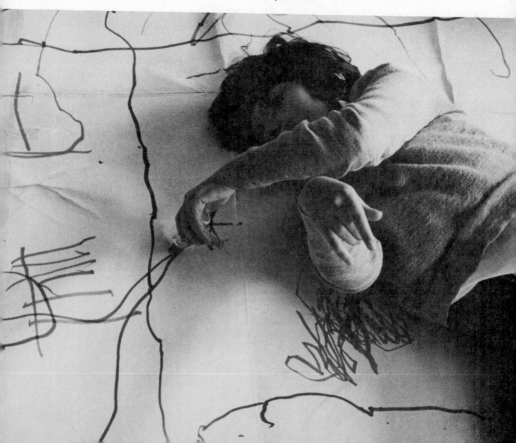

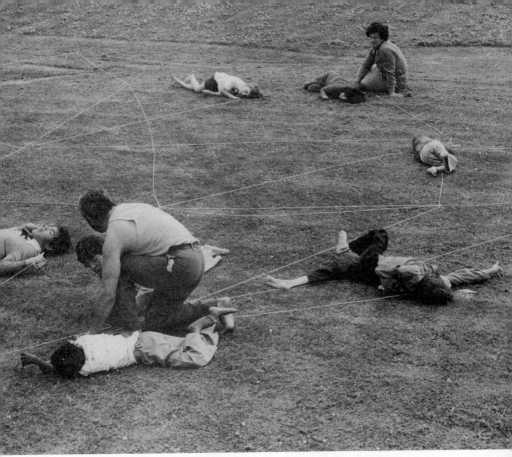

Taking a line for a walk at the Dame Hannah Rogers School

Photo by Bruce Kent

The project is undertaken in the belief that even those children and young people who have a handicap can enjoy and benefit from experience in the arts, and are often capable of high levels of achievement. The project is thus, by definition, concerned not only with the promotion of arts activity within the education of the handicapped, but with a striving towards quality of expression and perception.

Although it is rather early to make statements about the way this project is shaping, I think a comment is worthwhile on the work of my two colleagues who are exploring art, movement and vocal sound.

Bruce Kent and Keith Yon undertake experimental work at the Dame Hannah Rogers School for Cerebral Palsied Children. Some interesting ways of combining arts activities are being found. Children are encouraged to travel along the ground making marks around their bodies and marks to show various routes and modes of travel. These marks are all retained on a huge sheet of paper used finally as a mural. In another activity, movement on a lawn is tracked by stakes and string; this produces a fascinating three dimensional "sculpture." Other interesting relationships between modelling and speech come through explorations with dental plaster and shortbread mixture. By these activities the children can see mouth and teeth shapes, both enjoying the modelling activity and learning about themselves. Polystyrene blocks are also used for manipulation and moving with various structures built by the children. The activities aim, amongst other things, to improve body awareness, body centre and voice placing.

Although in its infancy, this threefold arts project — art, movement and music — hopes to produce evidence of beneficial activities for handicapped children. Not only does it aim to show how the arts can combine and inter-relate, but also how a wide variety of provision can offer choices to children who are variously handicapped.

REFERENCE
1. *Hearts and Hands and Voices*. David Ward. Oxford University Press 1976.

10

What Does Shape Do?

GINA LEVETE

Q. *You initiated the concept and organisation of Shape. The name conveys the idea of movement or dance but is there more to the work which is carried out?*

Shape is a link service between artists of every discipline and creatively deprived areas of the community, whether in an institution or a day centre, whether for the elderly or handicapped in hospital or for children in special schools or clubs. Its aim is to introduce creative arts activities wherever they will provide enjoyment and stimulation, as well as helping to break down any barriers of communication that may exist.

Any doubts as to the need have been quickly dispelled. Shape has been in existence for over four years. Already there are five similar operative regional services and three more under consideration. These work in co-operation with the Regional Arts Associations. It is far better for each region to meet its own needs with local talent; to translate the seed of the Shape idea into how it will best serve a locality. When asked about the overall purpose of Shape my answer is: "To allow people opportunities to enjoy themselves creatively." The response to the many varied activities and performances which Shape has linked together shows this to be so.

Young blind people meet together once a week after work to make and practice on the steel pans, and their steel band has become very professional. Another group of unsighted people are in their third year of a modern dance course. Art and leatherwork sessions for problem drinkers; poetry for the aged; creative writing, music and puppetry workshops in penal institutions; dance and drama sessions for the physically and mentally handicapped; drumming in an Intermediate Treatment centre; improvisation for young homeless and multi-racial groups—these are but a few of the regular workshop sessions that happen in and around London. Entertainments are also organised—music hall for the aged; folk and classical music performances in hospitals for the terminally ill; dance, jazz, reggae, mime and theatre groups perform to people who are unable to get out to public performances.

Q.   *Your work commenced in hospitals but has even ventured into prisons. What is the type of work and the response?*

We probably do more workshops than performances but the demand for performances from prisons throughout England and Wales has been very varied. They have asked for music performances, particularly with ethnic groups performing, poetry/folk evenings, some short plays, and both ethnic and contemporary dance. As for hospitals we have so far concentrated on poetry, folk and music, although music hall is very popular. In hospitals for the terminally ill it is usually classical music rather than pop or jazz.

I think that when artists first go to perform in a prison, they are slightly apprehensive. But the enormous warmth and the kind of feedback they get, as well as what they actually give to their audiences, is enormously beneficial. I think that this is something that all the artists working on a workshop basis say—that it gives an extra dimension to their professional work—to perform or work with a different group of people, probably a group of people they would never perform before or work with normally. This actually gives them ideas and makes them more creative for the work that they are doing most of the time. There is an incredible demand from all over the country. At first, I think, it comes from the imagination of the staff in both places. Through the very small amount of creative arts that have been introduced into these settings, people are increasingly realising that this is a wonderful way of breaking down barriers and encouraging communication between different groups of people. There is a sort of common denominator that everybody will enjoy something which also prevents the feeling of isolation that people who are institutionalised particularly have. To be creative or to watch something can often replace a pill.

We were always under the impression that the prisons and the Home Office were less than imaginative, but it is quite wrong. The Home Office gave Shape permission to introduce any kind of creative performance into any prison throughout England provided the Governor of that

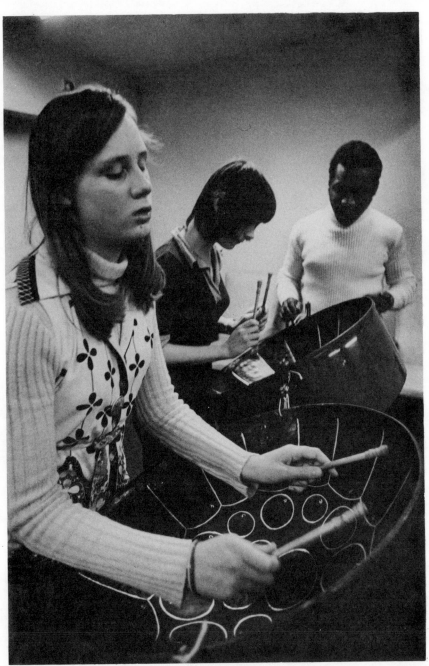

Members of the Sunsetters, a visually handicapped steel band, assisted by Shape

Photo by Chris Schwarz

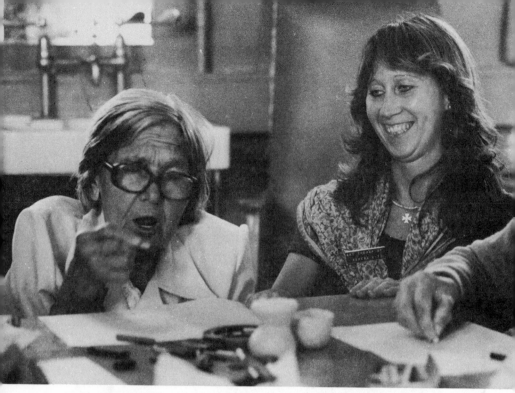

Artist Theresa Witz in a visual art workshop with elderly patients in a West London hospital ward

Photos by Chris Schwarz

A group of children finding new ways of expressing themselves and having fun through drama

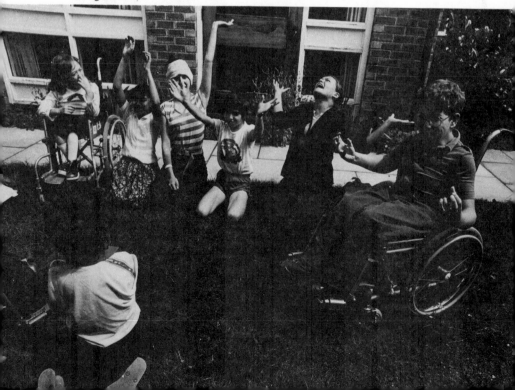

particular prison wanted it. So we sent out questionnaires asking what they would like in the way of arts, and replies were so varied – poetry workshops, creative writing, music, poetry/folk performances, puppetry, ethnic dance. You can no longer think that they are just people who can't see anything further than perhaps a nice classical music performance which can't offend anyone. They want things which the men and women can relate to.

I use dance to work with women in Holloway prison and I know that they do write a lot. I think that when you are in a situation where you are at a very low ebb, and I know myself, if you can write somehow it just keeps you from going right underground. In a situation like this where you are shut away from people, to be able to express yourself, to be able to write and to say your thoughts in the form of poetry, is one way of having an outlet.

We have asked the Home Office if they would consider allowing an anthology of poems written in British prisons to be collected and edited by someone, and they are considering the request at the moment. I have just come back from the USA where there is a similar organisation to Shape, only much bigger because it has far more money. They have prepared three anthologies of poems, written in prisons in New York and throughout the State, which have been tremendously popular. They are preparing another anthology now because of the success. Some very beautiful work comes from this kind of writing, from this kind of situation.

Q. *This seems to have the emphasis on recreation or entertainment rather than on therapy. Presumably there is no special therapeutic aim?*

Shape as a whole uses professional artists, and not therapists, who are interested in working in these areas as well as doing their own professional work. But it is therapeutic in that it gives people an outlet. For example, we have a West Indian who is teaching a group of young blind people how to form a steel band. We had some pans specially made by a West Indian which are slightly raised so that it is easier to feel the surface. This is something which you could say is therapeutic, because here we have a group of young people who are blind, getting together and wanting to form a steel band. Through this, I think, they will feel there is a sort of continuity and communication between them. Perhaps they wouldn't have all met up if it hadn't been for this, and if they are really good, they can perform like anyone else.

Q.   *There must be a major difficulty with finance if the*
     work extends as an introductory free service?

This arts project serves a wide area of the community and has exciting potential. For this reason both the Arts Council and the DHSS have now given Shape small grants. However, the main part of Shape's funding still has to come from the generosity of charitable foundations. Shape will always need both public and private funding. It has basically to be a free service to the community. Artists are paid a fee, as in any other of their working situations. When an activity is introduced to an institution or group on a regular weekly basis, Shape may fund the artist for the first three months. This allows untried activities and their potential to be assessed by artists and staff responsible in the appropriate setting before the organisation commits itself to taking over financial responsibility. In the main the organisations have managed to do this from various funding sources. Contributions are requested from the organisers initially towards a performance fee, but this should never inhibit the initial experiment so that the organisation and its members can experience the value of the arts activity. Before Shape commenced there was a gap of communication between the arts world and many small pockets of the community. Shape tries very hard to provide a service that will handle any request sensitively and quickly and ensure that the activity or performance of a professional standard will give maximum pleasure. It really is all to do with having fun.

NOTE:
Gina Levete has now left Shape to write and work freelance, and the new Director is Seona Reid.

11

Training and Therapeutic Services

LYNN ESKOW

Q. *The use of the arts with a distinct and direct aim of therapy is very different from the wider recreational purpose. How do you see the differences and needs of training?*

I represent two separate organisations, Sesame and the British Institute for the Study of the Arts in Therapy. As Co-ordinator of the Institute I would like to present that group's point of view regarding the training of professionals who work with sick and handicapped people through the Arts.

Sesame has been in existence since 1964. Its work is solely with the use of drama and movement in therapy. The Institute was established in 1978 under the sponsorship of Sesame; its interests are with all of the major art forms, when used for therapeutic purposes. The Institute has three primary concerns:

1. support for the establishment and maintenance of the highest possible standards for those who use any of the arts in a therapeutic setting;
2. provision of opportunities for ongoing study of the full implications of arts therapy;
3. creation of closer ties between the fields of art and health care.

Its membership is composed of recognised practising artists, educators, and qualified therapists in the visual arts, music, drama, movement and writing. In addition a panel of distinguished specialists from the fields of mental health and medicine serves in an advisory capacity.

I should like to make a few observations about the special responsibilities that are encountered by the artist when he/she begins to work with individuals or groups in therapeutic settings. The artist often has a view of life that is particularly fresh and vital. He may perceive the world with a sense of wonder and find newness all around, where the non-artist sees only the old and familiar. When the artist is able to bring his special vision and vitality to the non-artist, when he can help others to work in a satisfying way within an art form, then there is no question of the substantial contribution that he is making to their lives. Good teachers have been doing this for a very long time; encouraging their students to find their own ways of authentic expression through writing, music, the visual arts, drama, dance and movement. It is only fairly recently, however, that society has come to recognise the special importance of these kinds of activities for the men, women and children who are living in the community or in institutions with some form of serious illness or handicap. The growing awareness of the value of the creative arts for these people is to be applauded. And the provision of arts experiences for them is to be encouraged. I would like to suggest, however, that the awareness must be deepened and that the nature of the experiences provided must be carefully studied. We need programmes of continuous research into the effects of therapeutic arts activities, and rigorous training programmes for those wishing to undertake this work.

The artist is often intuitive and subjective in his creative life. These are his special strengths, for they enable him to persevere in his artistic work, often in the face of a discouraging lack of understanding or support from society. But what happens when the artist moves out of his own world of self-expression and enters into the world of other people's self-expression, taking on the role of teacher, therapist, enabler, or whatever label you may wish to use? He may not wish (or be able) to stand apart from his personal artistic intuition and his subjectivity. If he has not been trained, he may not understand the need to adjust one's own artistic standards and inclinations in order to suit the limitations and special problems of the people with whom he is asked to work. If he is not even aware of their limitations and special problems, it is unavoidable that he will make errors of judgment. Some of these errors can be extremely serious.

A great many people in the general community are afraid to even try to express themselves artistically because they are so fearful of self-exposure and failure. Sometimes, in a supportive environment, the resistance of these people can be overcome and they can find the encouragement they need in order to attempt something of an artistic nature. Often this proves extremely rewarding but, if improperly handled, it can result in the individual experiencing a sense of defeat and humiliation great enough to haunt and inhibit him for years. As a child, I experienced this with music; perhaps some readers can recall similar episodes.

There are countless stories to illustrate the ways in which well-intentioned but untrained (or insufficiently trained) people have inadvertently caused considerable distress to patients. These mistakes are made both by people working in the field of health who do not understand the creative process and by artists who do not understand the psychological implications of their actions. I would like to tell you about one incident which came to my attention when it was described at a public meeting last year in London. An artist was telling the audience about various arts activities that he had been able to find support for in his area hospitals. He showed slides of children's wards that had been beautifully and imaginatively decorated for the patients; paintings that had been displayed in the corridors; and sculpture in the gardens. He then went on to say that he had obtained the services of a friend of his, a poet who volunteered to come into the hospital to do a reading of his own work on one of the wards. Slides were shown of the event. One could see the poet and a fairly large group of patients in wheelchairs. The speaker said that the major work on the programme was a poem describing the wonders of childbirth and its great significance, both as a real and a symbolic act. "It was not," he said, "until after the conclusion of the programme that we learned that about eighty per cent of the patients were women who had just had abortions. But," he went on to add reassuringly, "none of the patients seemed to be at all upset, and many of them said how beautiful they had found the poem."

I don't know which aspect of this story distresses me most: the fact that no one had felt it necessary to inquire in advance about the kinds of patients who would be present; the very strong probability that there were some deep and painful reactions to the poem; or the fact that neither the speaker nor the poet apparently realised the significance of what had happened, even after being told about the history of the women in the group, and that one or two verbal reassurances seemed to settle the matter. There is no doubt at all in my mind that the people responsible for the poetry reading acted out of kindness and a desire to do something that would bring pleasure into the lives of the patients. But "love is not enough."

This incident illustrates another important point: the need for the artist, whether he is functioning as a performer, teacher, or therapist, to know how to recognise non-verbal signs of distress, which often contradict what is expressed through language. In my judgment, it also emphasises the fact that the artist has special responsibilities, even when he does not claim to be engaged in teaching or therapy. In this case the

82 *The Arts and Disabilities*

patients were not only an audience. How much greater, then, is the responsibility of the artist when the group is actively participating in the art experience!

> Q. *It would be an impossible task to train all artists and teachers in the whole theory of therapy. Can we not distinguish between the aims?*

It is sometimes difficult to make clear distinctions between therapy and teaching, between teaching and rehabilitative work, between recreation and social group work, and between other closely related fields. Obviously, activities in all of this work overlap in many ways, although the primary objectives of each discipline may be identifiably different. It is only when he is aware of the similarities and differences of these related disciplines that the professional can understand the need for remaining essentially within his own field of specialisation. Each of these fields provides a particular kind of training. It is unwise for the professional to ignore the differences in training and be tempted to move into a neighbouring area of professional responsibility, for which he has not been prepared, simply because the opportunity is there.

I don't think that many of us would knowingly get on to a bus in Central London with a driver who had never been in city traffic before, or entrust his child to a teacher who had read a lot of books but knew nothing about teaching or children. Surely the people whose interests and needs are our concern deserve, in all major aspects of their lives, the same kind of expertise that we expect from bus drivers and teachers. And, clearly, we consider the arts to be a major part of life for them, or we would not be considering the needs.

There is agreement amongst all of the leaders in arts therapy who are members of the Institute, that optimally anyone carrying out participatory arts activities in a therapeutic setting would be qualified in the following ways:

1 . He would understand the impact of arts experiences upon the person who is not accustomed to expressing himself artistically, and he would be aware that spontaneous art expression enables the individual to release what has been repressed and to discover previously unrecognised aspects of himself. (If this is not understood, participants may be subjected to feelings that are extremely difficult for them to handle, and serious damage may result. Equally, important opportunities for helping the individual may go unnoticed.)

2 . He would be extremely cautious about offering any interpretation of the patient's work to the patient himself, knowing that the patient may not be ready to verbalise his problem or to be confronted with it in a direct manner.

3 . He would understand what the individual might be saying about himself through his artistic expression, and its significance in relation both to that individual's particular needs and to his general illness or handicap. This requires knowledge about the overall problem (such as depression, schizophrenia or subnormality) and as much understanding as possible of the individual patients. Highly developed observation skills are necessary, for there are no formulae that can provide quick answers or necessarily valid interpretations.

4 . He would be thoroughly familiar with the art form he is using, objective about his own artistic involvement when he is with an individual or group and able to intuitively select the kinds of activities and experiences that are needed by the participants at any given moment. If an individual's behaviour seemed to indicate that he was having difficulty coping, the leader or therapist would know how to redirect him, gently and by means of the art experience, into a more secure state. Conversely, if the individual appeared ready to move ahead to a more difficult task, the therapist would know how to help him do so within the art form.

5 . He would understand that interfering with a patient's work by making value judgments about it or by offering suggestions about how it might be "improved" could seriously impair the patient's progress by curtailing his willingness or ability to express himself freely. It could also destroy the trust which is so necessary in the relationship between patient and leader.

6 . He would recognise the fact that the relationship between patient and leader, or therapist, is of paramount importance, for it is the leader or therapist's understanding of the patient's needs, his ability to accurately assess the patient's readiness for certain kinds of experiences, his appropriate responses to the patient's work, his warmth and support, and his professional objectivity that will enable the patient to move forward.

7 . The leader or therapist would have enough maturity and self-awareness not to project his own needs and feelings on to the patient, He would understand the therapeutic process sufficiently well to know when the patient might be projecting and when transference might be taking place. And he would know how to cope with these situations in the most helpful ways possible for the patient.

Clearly, these are skills and levels of understanding that are not quickly attained, and the Institute advocates long and thorough training for those whose work has therapeutic potential and responsibility. Further, we believe that arts therapy contributes to the healing process in a highly specialised way and that the therapist or leader should know how his work relates to the total treatment plan. We look forward to the day when arts therapists will serve as members of the therapeutic team.

Not everyone engaged in bringing arts activities to sick and handicapped people would consider his work to be at the depth that I have suggested, and the tendency might be for some to dismiss what has been said about training as not applicable to them. I would only reiterate the instance of the poem about childbirth, and point out that ignorance of the possible effects of mishandled arts experiences is no defence against them. We do not have the right to take risks of this kind with the people who are entrusted to our care. We must educate ourselves and our colleagues to the point where unnecessary risks will not be taken.

All of us who work through the arts do so because of a very deeply held belief that experience in an art is a basic need for everyone. And those of us who use the arts in therapeutic settings and special centres are convinced that they can enrich the quality of life and that, properly handled by trained and experienced people, they can have strong healing effects.

The artist whose life has been significantly enriched by his art understands its power in a way that the non-artist cannot. He often has a way of perceiving life and the world around him that is less bound by the constraints of convention than is the vision of the non-artist. He is usually quite inner-directed and has vitality. These are extremely valuable attributes for someone working with the sick and the handicapped; they place the artist in a unique starting point for this work. It remains, however, only a starting point.

NOTE:

Lynn Eskow has since returned to work in the USA. The new Co-ordinator of BISAT is Mrs M. Attlee.

12

Conclusions for the Future

HENRY WALTON

Q. *As a psychiatrist and with a life-long interest in the arts, do you have a special view of Life and Art?*

People differ greatly in their response to art. For certain people, aesthetic experience is at the centre of their lives. For very many other people art in its various forms can enhance their existence and immeasurably improve the quality of their life. That still leaves the large numbers of people, who may not actively seek regular stimulus from music or painting or drama or literature—but they nevertheless benefit from the unobtrusive influence of these art forms on their lives, no matter how much attenuated or altered. Through the newspapers, on gramophone records, on posters, on the radio and on television, current art forms profoundly contribute to the spirit of the times, and bear on the social climate in which we pass our lives.

A person's response to any form of art is highly complex, and as yet only partially understood. A range of attitudes and reactions is involved in the response to a work of art: a receptive mood, some degree of self-surrender, and often an inner experience which can be strong enough to diminish one's awareness of other present realities. The person largely forgets about the self as well, while responding to a work of art—a play, a painting, a novel, or a musical work. A feature of the aesthetic experience appears to be this partial loss of self, one's attention claimed, in a state of intensified awareness, by the work of art to which one responds.

Q. *How do you transfer this opinion to the experiences of the disabled?*

The two seminars at Dartington and Stirling made it imperative to explore further whether disabled people are greatly more cut off from contact with art than they need be. The conclusion of such inquiry will almost certainly confirm that disabled people are unjustifiably deprived of artistic experience. For an entire realm of significant experience to be inaccessible to disabled people is wholly unacceptable. The public intention in a civilised society, when conditions are favourable enough, to provide all people with the necessities of life, must now extend to reducing the barriers obstructing the disabled from access to the arts.

Only neglect, and lack of imagination, prevents a great many disabled people, both in the community and in institutions such as hospitals, from receiving the special help which will enable them more readily to visit exhibitions, see plays and hear concerts in the customary public places. Very many more disabled people than is the case at present must be enabled to benefit from scientific progress which has made books more accessible to the blind, and music more audible to some deaf people.

The inquiry which ought to follow needs to take account of the specific type of the disability present, and the age of the person at the onset of the disability. A life-long affliction has very different consequences for a person than a similar disability incurred later in life. A person who is already adult when becoming disabled will have the incalculable assets of a developed personality and completed skills. We may consider it critically important that somebody already aware and responsive to an art form when disability strikes should be enabled to resume enjoyment of it again, to the extent still feasible despite the impairment of mind or body resulting from the damaging accident or illness. In addition, many of those who have the affliction of life-long handicap may also prove capable, when their remaining ability is studied with ingenuity, of greater response to certain forms of art than is recognised at present.

There can be no doubt following the two seminars that very considerable development is called for in art therapy of many forms, at present scarcely heeded. Far too little organised action has followed the frequent demonstrations of the benefits provided when musicians and actors perform in hospitals, and the humanising effect on the hospital's atmosphere when good paintings customarily hang on the walls and regular exhibitions by painters are arranged. Art is too meagrely and too sporadically brought into hospitals for the chronically disabled, and that neglect occurs in spite of the readiness to assist on the part of the artists concerned.

As serious has been the inattention to the benefit that artists, through the medium of their artistic ability, can provide for the disabled. There is a close connection between physical and emotional stability and between concentration and the focussing of strength. The artists who have succeeded in finding such therapeutic scope have demonstrated that patients can be enabled, however rudimentarily, to paint, to dance, to act, or to be musical. At times the disability at issue may be formidable enough to daunt all but the most intrepid instructor, but the artists who have persevered, sometimes in the face of official discouragement, have made it possible for many disabled people to respond in a way not previously possible. An instance is when a psychiatric patient by means of painting manages to convey depths of experience which could not be expressed verbally; such artistic activity may enable the patient to escape damaging isolation and engage in a shared experience with others.

The two seminars clearly showed the directions which future effort must now take. Different participants may well have valued some aspects of the meetings above others, depending on individual interests and responsibilities. Everybody present will have been alive to remarkable elements in the meetings which, viewed in conjunction, signal the considerable possibilities that can be developed in the future.

In the first place, many exceptional people now working with disabled people gave demonstrations of their special abilities. We saw talented practitioners who sometimes astonished the audience by their originality and boldness. They were singularly devoted, painstaking, persistent and effective in what they sought to do. They had modified and adapted their art form—whether painting, dancing, music or drama—to make it applicable to the disabled, and in most instances to enable the disabled to take a direct part in it themselves. Children with substantial handicap were actively encouraged or disarmingly manhandled through sequences of movement, impossible for them without external assistance, to their evident enjoyment; physical contact was provided for them with their instructors or other assistants, the latter sometimes disabled like them, as in the case of deaf actors. We were shown only too clearly why "bodies are the best equipment." In the hands of these teachers the customary taboo against touching was set aside; close physical contact was accepted and altogether justified by the new movements and additional forms of awareness initiated. The deaf were helped to mime, with verbal and musical accompaniments being supplied when sound was not in their own capacity. The experts enabled the participants in the Seminars to understand and actually witness how they went about applying their particular art form in the setting provided for them in their work.

Q. *We both gained an impression that artists in various disciplines were unaware of developments in other parts of the country or in other artistic disciplines.*

It did not escape the participants either how unfortunate and sometimes damaging was the isolation in which many of the experts worked. In the

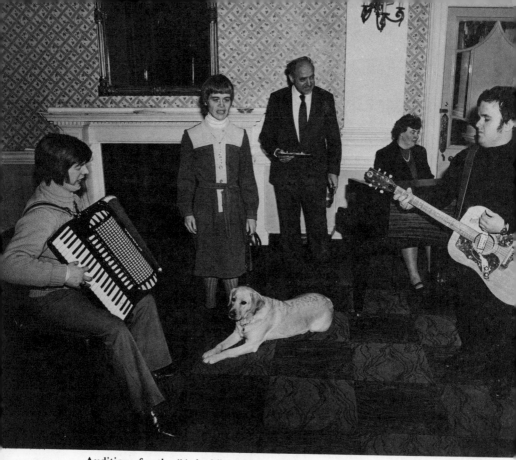

Auditions for the "Aeleph" project with Leonard Friedman whereby musicians who are disabled will play in concert with the Scottish Baroque Ensemble

Photo by courtesy of BBC Scotland

same art fields practitioners of similar interests worked unknown to one another, despite the obvious advantages that would follow from a shared endeavour. Moreover, if experts in a particular field can be made properly aware about activities in other art sectors, all forms of art therapy stand to gain considerably. Among the different forms of art used, there are common features in the approaches and the styles of experts, which should be generally known across the boundaries of the separate art forms. Programmes and procedures inevitably have at least some features which are mutually relevant. Another great benefit, to be expected from improved contact across the boundaries segregating the different art forms, is the stimulus one expert can gain from witnessing another at work; whether or not they practise a similar artistic activity, there will be common ingredients in the therapeutic effect of the artists. We already know what the factors are that beneficially influence handicapped or disturbed people. Among these, meaningful contact with another person, the arousing of hope, and the mobilisation of competence are prominent. All three of these factors can be mobilised in art therapy.

Some artists, as is to be expected in view of their unusual personal qualities, work best in relative isolation. Nevertheless, the seminars left us in no doubt that artists have profound contributions to make to the members of staff of hospitals and to many helping professionals responsible for the disabled. Any artists working in the institution must be known and their work must be visible to other members of staff. Now that the Department of Health officially accepts artists on the staff of institutions (making the initial proposal, now under further discussion, that they might be affiliated with Occupational Therapy departments), artists can have an important influence in the institution as a whole. Their influence may liberate members of staff to some extent from routine and convention, and help them to learn new procedures which can transform their own professional work. For this to occur, hospital staff must be drawn to collaborate with artists where appropriate, and be given some instruction about the art form being used for therapy of the disabled. A psychiatrist, for example, should not merely appreciate the obvious enhancement of experience provided for his patients by an art therapist; in addition, he should be shown and pay attention to the actual paintings as well, for the relevance of these works to his treatment and their significance for his patients.

Q. *You obviously valued the discussions and demonstrations, but was there any unusual feature for you?*

Another fact emerged that made my experience as chairman of the Stirling meeting both engrossing and challenging: the extent and range of talents possessed by the participants *not* featured in the programme. As the meeting proceeded, the contributors from the audience made it evident that the experts — often unknown to them, as I have already indicated — had numerous counterparts present, participants of unusual ability, often with an unsuspected range of experience. These gifted and experienced members of the audience appreciated instantly what the artists were attempting as they explained their own work with the disabled. Members of the audience could report equivalent projects, and at times amplify the contribution of the experts.

A final important lesson for the future became clear. The meetings served to bring together many artists working in related fields who, collectively, gave ample grounds for confidence that art increasingly can be made accessible to the disabled, and has an important place in individual and social rehabilitation. Artists can greatly assist handicapped people, and art can help to improve the fate of the disabled. There are many artists who are equipped and ready to help, if only they are given the support and facilities they need for the task.

Fortunately, the setting up of the Scottish Committee on Arts and Disability is now such a facility, funded in a unique manner by the Royal Bank, the Scottish Arts Council and the Carnegie Trust. This is a sound beginning to assist the work of disabled artists. A concert by them in association with the Scottish Baroque Ensemble is already arranged for the International Year of Disabled People. In addition, artists are being encouraged to work in a range of institutions and we are witnessing in Scotland a new awareness amongst organisations arranging courses in participatory arts and crafts.

I know that discussions are taking place with the Arts Council of Great Britain for a national inquiry into the whole subject and this should highlight actual work, needs and resources for the decade. This is an encouraging sign.

Appendix

ARTICLES RELATING TO DISCUSSIONS
AT THE SEMINARS

Disability ?

CLAUDIA FLANDERS

Q. *You were married to an outstanding entertainer who was disabled, and you have worked voluntarily with and for disabled people. At Stirling you introduced discussion on the problems of access. What are your feelings?*

You may remember the little song which my late husband, Michael, liked to use in ending his *At the Drop of a Hat* show — it was part of the "Lord Chamberlain's Regulations" which he and Donald Swann had set to music, and it contained those dreadful lines, "all gangways, passageways and staircases . . . must be kept entirely free . . . of chairs . . . or any other obstruction!" It's a pity that, some twenty-two years after that song was first performed, most people who are severely disabled are forced to discuss how they are going to get *out* of a theatre or cinema hall long before they even arrive at the performance!

I once mentioned in an article which was published in the Edinburgh *What's On* magazine, that while theatre managements would go to any lengths to get Michael in to do his work (such as using a block and tackle in Aberdeen!), he was considered to be just as much of a "safety hazard," so to speak, if he came along merely as a spectator.

It is true that managements are still using the idea of Safety Regulations to cover their worries and fears about disabled people, but I like to think that Michael in his particular life and work did something very special in the way of breaking down such barriers. People who had previously believed that they could not spend even ten minutes, let alone two hours, with a person in a wheelchair without feeling in some way very disturbed, found to their amazement that they learned to forget all about his disability — in less than ten minutes. . . .

I feel that people who have experienced physical disability through accident or illness usually have more to teach than to learn. That is, there is something about what they have gone through or — in the case of progressive disease — are preparing to go through, which enriches their thought in a way which we can only begin to fathom. Surely the learning process which has already taken place is a very profound one? I might go further and say that I wonder whether teaching and therapy can even make a good start at all without a learning and listening effort by the teacher.

> Q.   *What can we learn so as to encourage imaginative opportunities to reduce any aspect of a condescending approach and to understand the view of the disabled person?*

There is an enormous amount to learn about the many avenues being opened for teaching those with a disability, particularly in the field of the arts. It might be of help if I mention a few of my husband's general lines of thought about working and living, and then to list briefly a few of the practicalities of his professional life.

It is hard to realise now, but once upon a time Michael was considered well-nigh unemployable. Even today his DHSS file carries the qualification, "100% disabled." He only got his first radio job because he finally managed to teach the BBC that a person could take part in a radio programme by speaking into a microphone sitting down! One factor which helped Michael—as it does so many—was that special inner intensity which can colour the attitude of a disabled person who is mentally fit enough to keep on trying. Michael told me, when he was describing his polio disaster at 21, that after you have been through the moment when you know you are terribly close to death, everything that follows—life itself—is a "gift." "It's borrowed time," he said, "and you have to use it." I think that in teaching as well as in learning, people have to find a vein of gold, if you like, a special resource which can be turned to advantage; and Michael seemed throughout his life to be able to find his own resource and to help others to use theirs.

When audiences laughed, for example, they were partly laughing at what Michael had shown up inside *their* minds. Using their imagination was the key to their enjoyment. But every audience was new and different from night to night and country to country—Michael always treated them as individuals.

In fact, the right of all people, able-bodied and handicapped alike, to consider themselves unique and be considered unique by those around them, was central to Michael's thinking. He rejected generalisations—as most of us would claim to do—and particularly disapproved of the way assumptions are so often made about people with a disability, as if they were part of some definable group. Even after thirty-two years in a wheelchair Michael found himself continually treated as if he were not only unable to walk but deaf and mentally retarded as well; and people, if they helped at all, were still failing to listen to a single word of instructions as to *how* to help him. . . .

But if he believed in people's uniqueness, there was also a sting in the tail: Michael did not believe that all people were necessarily uniquely interesting, or talented: "I reserve the right," he remarked once, "to hate everybody, regardless of race, creed or political belief!" Michael excused no-one—not children, neurotics or even his wife's relations!—for ineptitude, bad judgment or being just plain boring. . . . Yet he was warm and genuine in his appreciation of beauty and excellence, wherever he found them. Conversely, however, he made no special allowances: I fear that Michael would have thought a violin played badly, sounded just as bad whether or not the player was disabled. He might have proved rather a tough customer at any seminar!

Summing up, I think I should refer to the note I found in one of Michael's diaries: "Motto: if it's WORTH DOING, DO IT WELL!" He could, at the height of his career, honestly say that what he was doing, he was doing well. Yet he was always teaching as well as entertaining, though his fans never knew it.

Comments from Dartington

BILL SEARY

Q. *From your background, what were your main impressions of the Dartington discussions?*

In Dartington I started by saying a little bit about myself in order to set my remarks in context and it is probably right that I do the same now. I work for the National Council of Voluntary Organisations in an administrative capacity. Such paper qualifications as I have are in the physical sciences. A lack of skills or qualifications in either the arts or the caring professions might seem to reduce my ability to comment on the Dartington Seminar in an intelligent way, but it does give me a certain neutrality and it helps to explain why I take a fairly down-to-earth line in looking for practical results which could be of use to disabled people.

What follows is really in three parts. First is an attempt to collect together some of the underlying themes of the weekend: second come some ideas for future action, and last are some comments on the seminar itself which I hope will assist the preparation of a further seminar. I apologise to any participant who feels that her or his contribution has been pirated or ignored: there is no intention to do either.

As at all gatherings, there emerged some areas of broad agreement and some areas where questions were raised rather than answered.

I have identified four matters of agreement and three matters of doubt. It must be a mark of the skill with which the programme was put together that all the issues were raised directly or indirectly by Cherry Vooght in her opening talk and were in our minds for the whole seminar.

Agreements

(i) Any activity contemplated as an "Art for the Benefit or Care of the Disabled" must be enjoyable. The fun of the activity is a very real part of its value.

(ii) Human relations are fundamental. Trust between the leader and the client produces a fruitful, caring relationship.

(iii) The experience of life that the leader has at his or her disposal is as important as any paper qualifications.

(iv) The trend towards the identification of more and more specialities is useful. This, however, has to be qualified by the need to share experiences across the boundaries of specialities. Little boxes are all right, you could say, provided they have doors and windows.

Q. *Matters of discussion or doubt seem to centre around role. What were three main issues which you identified?*

There is a whole spectrum of concept — Therapy, Teaching, Entertainment — behind the activities described at the seminar. This covers those who are actively looking to alter a patient's condition, those who are trying to develop a person, and those who just want to bring a bit of enjoyment into the lives of disadvantaged people. Naturally, it is very difficult for participants with such a diversity of motivations to reach agreement. Those who are interested in therapy place much emphasis on training in order to reduce the risk of doing damage. Those who are interested in entertainment place more emphasis on spontaneity. Teachers can try to square this circle by stressing the role of care workers in addition to the teacher. Perhaps it is useful here to make particular mention of the limited range of arts and of disabilities that were under discussion. I have a feeling that a seminar with the same title that concentrated on plastic arts for physically handicapped adults would not have been so concerned with these issues. Perhaps the wisest words came from one of the discussion groups — "no one can work alone: no one can cover all aspects."

One of the problems raised, particularly by people from the organisations concerned with disabled people, was that it was not easy to recruit leaders for arts activities. Obviously, the existence of Shape is some sort of answer but its capacity is limited, particularly outside London.

A related but rather different point arose in connection with helpers. Nearly all the techniques described at the seminar depended upon a supply of friendly, sympathetic but not necessarily skilled people to join in the activities. Rather little is said about them, however, and a number of questions arise. How are they recruited? Do such bodies as the National Federation of Women's Institutes or Community Service Volunteers have a role in this? Should they be paid? If so, at what sort of rate? What training do they need?

PHAB, who turn the whole thing round to make the relationship between the physically disabled person and the able-bodied the centre of their activities, apparently have difficulty in contacting sufficient disabled people to match the able-bodied participants, but this may be a rather special case because of their roots in the youth movement.

There seemed to me to be a number of issues in this area of "Them and Us" which never really came to the surface during the talks. These are perhaps best framed as challenging questions:

There was a certain amount of discussion of the divide between work and leisure. Yet for many mentally handicapped people who live in homes or hospitals there really is no such divide. How far can we use our own concepts of leisure when making plans for them? Our intention may be to provide disabled people with the same opportunities as the rest of us, but is there not a danger that we will be giving people little choice but to join in activities which only a minority of ordinary people choose to follow?

The use of movement and touch have been widely advocated as techniques of expression for handicapped people. No one has suggested, however, that we should have started the seminar with a movement session on the lawns of Dartington's courtyard. Are we misguided in hiding our own needs in this matter or presumptuous in imputing them to others?

We seem to have agreed that involvement with clients is a dangerous thing but that commitment to them is essential. What, however, is the difference between these? Where does the one become the other?

Q.   *What were the main suggestions which might answer*
some of these pertinent queries?

This is really a list of ideas that came up during the weekend:

(i) There should be an independent inquiry into the use of arts for the disabled. It should be reasonably comprehensive but, most important, obliged to report quickly.

(ii) There is a need for a national clearing house of information on arts for the disabled. This would depend heavily upon support from all the existing organisations.

(iii) Further seminars should be arranged; some of these should explore the questions raised this weekend, others could be used as an opportunity to demonstrate a range of techniques to people who might know of uses for them.

(iv) Regional Arts Councils should be invited to consider the contribution they could make to the availability of arts to the disabled people in their areas.

(v) Attention should be given to the needs of the 16+ group.

(vi) Prevention is better than a cure. The availability of help for people who are under stress must be a priority.

Q. *What were your overall conclusions?*

In thinking of this, I turned first to the stated aims that appeared on the programme:

> The purpose of the seminar is to allow leaders of organisations concerned with disability and the arts to review the main features of the various arts as recreation and as therapy when disabled persons are involved. Limitations of time do not allow all art forms to be illustrated, and the visual arts are excluded from this particular seminar, which is concerned primarily with leisure in the community.

The following comments should be seen as criticism which is meant to be constructive. This was a first attempt to discuss the issues and the meeting was of tremendous value in spreading awareness and showing what has been achieved. Future seminars will profit from the experience gained.

(i) With the exception of the Dartington project, all the work discussed has been in the broad area of drama and movement. It could be useful to widen this in future.

(ii) In hindsight it was probably unrealistic to expect to reach a consensus between the people mainly concerned with therapy and the others concerned with teaching or entertainment. A future seminar might profit from concentrating on one aspect or the other.

(iii) There was a noticeable absence of disabled people because invited organisations did not nominate a disabled representative. Some should certainly be involved in future gatherings.

(iv) There was not enough opportunity for people to discuss the information that was being supplied. Additional discussion group sessions some time in the middle of the seminar would have been useful.

(v) The range of skills and techniques discussed was wide and interesting. For many people the high point was Veronica Sherborne's film, but the organisers are to be congratulated on the way in which the entire programme fitted together.

In conclusion, we reached a broad agreement on fundamentals but left a host of questions for further study. We arrived and departed with the firm conviction that the range of facilities available should be the same for everyone, disabled or not.

Comments from Stirling

SUE INNES

Q. *The linking of the words "arts" and "disabled"
poses a challenge and problems. As an artist and
journalist how did you interpret the significant
features?*

The Stirling seminar spent most of its time looking at very specific art
forms with specific client groups. And this is no criticism — not only did it
illustrate the variety of possibilities but it also reminded us, as Claudia
Flanders said, that people are unique; there is no great value and there
can be harm in categorising — in "lumping together." Discussion after
each speaker's contribution had been concerned mainly with the
practical. Had this activity been used with disturbed children? Where did
the people come from for one-to-one work?

With a remit as broad as "Arts for the Benefit and Care of Disability"
generalisation is dangerous ground. Those people who have what we call
disabilities have widely varying needs, problems, abilities, aptitudes. The
arts are not easily lumped together either — rather we were talking of a
group of activities linked together by "family resemblance." The
possibilities must lie in some mathematical relationship between these
two categories! To define the value of the arts in relation to disability is
no easy task — though to demonstrate it was much easier. In the final
discussion these difficulties of definition began to be explored. Could a
whole community be described as disabled? Weren't we talking of needs
which we all had? I would answer yes, but some more urgently than
others.

Nonetheless — it seems possible to draw from the total multi-faceted
content a few threads which struck me as particularly important and
which have relevance to the theme.

Veronica Sherborne's work with movement with mentally
handicapped children: as well as the immediately apparent physical
values of increased co-ordination, suppleness, touching-ness, she drew
our attention to a progression in two ways — the progression in
relationships, from being receptive to the adult's direction, through

taking initiative in the pair and taking shared responsibility, to work with other children; and the progression in body awareness and self-awareness. "I have to join children up." In both these aspects it was clear that the results for the child were significant to the child's whole development. And this I think deepened, through demonstration rather than abstraction, the understanding that we were talking of much more than simply recreation or occupation. Her work also emphasised that:

"it must, above all, be fun" — a point which needs no amplification;

it is about relating to people, not objects — "people make the best apparatus";

and — a point made in later discussion — "we all have, to a greater or lesser degree, a taboo about touching, and this may be especially so in relation to the handicapped.

Joyce Laing set her work as an art psychotherapist in the context that "from the beginning of time people's well-being and the arts have been interwoven" — underlining again that we were not concerned with special provision for special people (though there are special aspects) but with needs we all have, and that to forget this could lead to a distortion in provision. She commented on the current search for identity, for meaning in life, for "a balancing of society's psyche." She emphasised, therefore, the growing importance of arts centres and art therapy. This again seemed a keypoint — that the implicit view of many organisations concerned with the social services and disability that the arts are "the icing on the cake" vastly minimises their importance. Or, as one artist put it, "I know that for me art is necessary . . . but just try getting a job as a dance therapist in the NHS." Art psychotherapy is important because "Art is a hot-line to the unconscious." The therapist must be an artist, someone who understands the language of imagery, and conversely if arts centres are to be a resource for the needy, then people with therapeutic skills must work in them. I took from this and from the commitment of other participants, the importance of the teacher, therapist or initiator being an artist, with a genuine involvement with the form, rather than someone who sees it as "good for you" or "fun for you."

It was interesting to note in the discussion afterwards the phrases, "speaking as a philistine . . ." "of course I'm a complete layman. . . ." Is art *so* separate and scarey a business?

Pat Keysell's work with the theatre of the deaf: the perspective was altered to an art not as therapy primarily, but very much as an art. The theatre of the deaf is based on the natural sign language of deaf people and it is therefore an art form which they can take to standards of excellence. This seemed to me a valuable example — it set an emphasis on what the handicapped person can *give*.

The discussion led by Claudia Flanders centred primarily on "access" — a simple but essential aspect of the arts and disability. We spoke of access in terms of being able easily and with dignity to get in and out of buildings (*and* in the event of fire), but also in the sense that people will feel able, encouraged and wanted to attend events, and in terms of the willingness of audiences to accept, e.g. a party of mentally handicapped people, next to them at the theatre. This latter point was seen as needing education and perseverance, but it was also suggested that handicapped people shouldn't have to so often go out in large, organised parties. The discussion also illustrated the sad fact that although it is very evident what needs to be done to make ease of access a reality, nonetheless it's *not* being done.

Claudia Flanders also highlighted the evident (but often ignored) need for the organisations concerned with disability to communicate, and to work in co-operation rather than competition.

Dorothy Heathcote wove a spell round her audience, increasing our own imaginative experience as she did so. Among the insights she contributed I was particularly struck by her saying that "you're a lucky person if you're living below the task level." This indicated to me the importance of seeing arts for disability as an opportunity rather than an occupation. There is the danger of devaluing what is happening and deflecting the individual's creative energy by seeing the activity as "make-work" or "time-filling." She also emphasised that the mentally handicapped people she works with may not find it easy to do the tasks we invent for them, but that they *can* function at the deeper, more meaningful level. "There is no truth known to man that is not available to the meanest of minds." Dorothy Heathcote also drew our attention to the preventive force of the "rule of law." "Oh we can't use the dining room because the staff have lunch then." "We always keep *that* windowsill clear." I wonder how many budding Dorothy Heathcotes, Veronica Sherbornes or Joyce Laings have been held back by rigidity and fear of the strange? There was a further reminder of the "easy" assumption — "there's very little appeal made to the skills, tenderness, authority, which they have"; and that education cannot be an imposition — it happens from the inside.

Alastair Pye brought attention back to a central theme: that music is great therapy for handicapped children because it's great therapy for us all. Two other particular points stand out: that *"you* can do it." He was eager to demonstrate that you don't have to be a musician to do useful work in this way, that to spread and develop this work didn't require expertise or cash, just willingness. This point was later taken up in discussion with the suggestion that we should look to see what present resources and ingenuity could provide in the way of developments. Alastair Pye also apologised for the quality of the pianos. What sort of thinking is it that assumes that a piano used with handicapped children doesn't need tuning?

Q. *Challenging thoughts! How do you view the challenge of the future?*

There was an element of "us and them," not helped by there being so few disabled people at the seminar (which I know was not because they were not invited but because organisations did not choose to send them). There was also something of the "we know what's good for you" disease. I have also noticed that many organisations concerned with the needs of disabled people are staffed at decision-making level by able-bodied people. At the same time they may campaign to increase employment for the disabled — this, too, when "self-help" is one of the most important trends in the social services. And so there is a need it seems for disabled people to have the opportunity to take over the running of these organisations, for a programme of positive discrimination to allow disabled people to overcome any handicaps which prevent them from doing so already.

Although the educational aspects of "art and disability" were much discussed, there was no discussion of the lack of opportunity for students in Scotland to learn the sorts of skills under discussion.

There were many groups of potential beneficiaries inevitably excluded because of the lack of time. I suspect that the elderly may not have come up anyway. But the over 70s include people who suffer from physical and mental illness, with the added handicap of poverty and often unwanted retirement. The types of art therapies discussed would be valuable to them.

And one final thought — the seminar generated enormous enthusiasm in its participants, as "talking shops" so often do not do. There were gathered together people (not in the least the representatives of the Scottish Arts Council) with the positions and the influences to *make things happen*. And we most of us were in a position to know of the need — of children whose lives are empty of stimulus and fun, whose potential for growth is not being met, of old people and mental patients in long-stay hospitals whose incapacity is being exacerbated by days spent in boredom and futility. The seminar will have its real meaning if we can keep alive that enthusiasm and if we are able to put into practice the ideas we discussed then.

NOTE:

Following the Stirling seminar a new project has been initiated in Scotland under the name of SCAD— the Scottish Committee for Arts and Disability—with a Project Leader and support staff to encourage and arrange performance and participation by disabled people, and to introduce artists into a range of institutions and centres for the disabled and disadvantaged.

The project is funded by the Royal Bank in association with the Scottish Arts Council and Carnegie UK Trust, with Henry Walton as Chairman of the voluntary committee.

Who Cares about the 5½%?

ROD FISHER

Q. *I know from your work at the Arts Council that you are concerned about the provision of the arts for handicapped people. How do you view the present situation?*

"Most people do not readily associate the arts with the handicapped. Or, when combining both, they think of recreation or art therapy. Despite the public's lack of awareness, there are and have been many handicapped professional artists — musicians, painters, dancers, playwrights, and artists who are blind, emotionally disturbed, deaf, crippled and retarded. Artists like these overcame their handicaps, but more important, they overcame or detoured around barriers that inhibited their involvement in arts activities which were accessible to non-handicapped people. Nevertheless, the vast majority of handicapped people still perceive the arts as an inconvenient obstacle course strewn with rules, regulations, revolving doors, and inaccessible opportunities." This quote from an American report, *Arts and the Handicapped — An Issue of Access,*[1] was expressing concern about the situation in the USA. The assessment could equally apply to Britain.

Estimates of the number of handicapped people vary according to the definition of disablement used. However, according to Amelia Harris' book *Handicapped and Impaired Persons in Great Britain*, there are over three million physically and mentally handicapped people in Britain, or something like 5½% of the population. It is a minority group, but as Lord Snowden said at the press launch of the International Year of Disabled People: "It is a shattering thought that in this country alone there are more people suffering from some kind of handicap than the alarming number of unemployed, who rightly are the subject of deep concern." Here are some three million fellow citizens who are entitled to exercise their right to participate in society to the full extent of their abilities. It is shameful, but true, that when it comes to enabling the handicapped to participate in or enjoy the arts, they continue to represent an area of serious neglect so far as arts agencies and arts providers are concerned.

When considering arts for the handicapped, many people fall into the conceptual trap of assuming that the activity will be provided as a diversion to audiences incapable of understanding it – the implication being that the institutionalised are somehow inferior to us. Others automatically equate arts provision for the impaired with therapy. Because of this it is important to stress that a clear distinction can be made between the use of art or creative activity as therapy on the one hand, and providing the opportunity for the handicapped to have access to professional artists and artistic experience on the other. Both are valid, but in my view they are different.

Michael Spencer, Executive Director of the American organisation Hospital Audiences Incorporated, which takes artists, writers and performers into rehabilitative settings, has described the distinction admirably: "The goal is to develop the usually untapped creative talents of those confined to these facilities . . . the emphasis is on enjoyment of the process, and developing pride in the product through its being shared with others within the institution, and increasingly, the outside world. One is cognisant that this activity might have other outcomes, which may, in part, be described as 'therapeutic', and also as . . . 'vocationally' oriented. . . . The development of skills in painting can lead to . . . relief of tension, anxiety and alienation generated by the institutionalisation, self-mastery and the strengthening of ego etc. However, all these artistic experiences are pursued with the goal of advancing the production and enjoyment of art. In this process, aesthetic (and not behavioural) criteria is employed. These are classes – 'education' if you so desire to call it – tailored to fit the context in which they are presented. They are not, by definition, arts therapy." And Spencer again: "As long as quality works of art are presented intact, even with the utmost attention to the secondary consideration of 'the therapeutics', is this not still, and foremost, an aesthetic or artistic experience, and not a session of therapy . . . ?"[2]

Staff at institutions frequently express genuine surprise at the obvious pleasure their "charges" derive from exposure to arts performances. Not that the value of the experience is confined to the handicapped recipient; professional artists often find that performing for disabled or disadvantaged people is especially rewarding. A leading actress of the Royal Shakespeare Company remarked after a performance of *Sylvia Plath* in a women's prison, that she had never before performed in a situation where the usual expectations and assumptions of an experienced theatre-going audience were not operative. She described it as both terrifying and artistically challenging. Certainly the artistic experience is no less valid because it is presented in an institutional setting rather than a theatre.

Q. *Can you tell me how the Arts Council supports the needs of disabled audiences and performers?*

The Council's involvement with arts provision specifically for the disabled is largely confined to its financial support of the work of Shape. Of course some of the arts companies in receipt of Council revenue subsidy or project grants, present performances for disabled audiences as part of their programme of activities. The Council also runs a scheme through which works of art are lent to hospitals. With regard to performers, the Council provides project support to the Interim Theatre Company, which comprises both hearing and deaf actors, and Terry Ruane, of Interim, has received a grant to study the techniques employed by the National Theatre of the Deaf in the USA.

When considering subsidy for disabled performers or groups, the Council is confronted by a fundamental philosophical difficulty. Traditionally, the Council's support for arts organisations is based on the artistic quality of their work; and while other factors, such as attendances, financial and administrative competence, the ability to raise money from other sources, and the balance between London and the regions, are taken into consideration, the criterion of standards is usually paramount. In any case some disabled performers would not expect to be judged any differently than their able-bodied counterparts. Nevertheless, the question arises, is it fair to expect the disabled to attain high artistic standards without some assistance which acknowledges their enormous disadvantages? It's a dilemma which the Council has not been able to resolve. However, as you know, the Council has intimated its readiness to support the Carnegie National Inquiry into Arts and Disability, which is bound to examine the arts needs of both handicapped performers and audiences. It is conceivable that some new Council initiatives will emerge in the light of that Committee's report.

Q. *What are the employment prospects for those disabled people wishing to pursue a career in the arts?*

Quite frankly, the opportunities for advancement are very poor. The performing arts world, for example, is highly competitive, and there is a ruthless pursuit of excellence. The small number of handicapped

performers who have achieved professional success have had to
overcome enormous obstacles; and remember, some of this select group,
like that excellent and courageous clarinettist, Alan Hacker, were already
established on successful professional arts careers when they were struck
by permanent illness or injury.

At a recent conference at Bulmershe College on "Higher Education
and Employment Opportunities for the Deaf," Michael Elliott, Chief
Administrator of the National Theatre, considered that deafness was an
"insuperable disqualification" for working in theatre. None of the four
major national arts companies—the Royal Opera House, English
National Opera, the Royal Shakespeare Company and the National
Theatre—have deaf people on their payrolls, although they do
occasionally engage a partially deaf or disabled performer for a specific
production. Furthermore, because the employment prospects are so
grim, drama schools frequently refuse entry to handicapped young
people. So disabled people cannot even acquire the skills to qualify for
the profession.

One way for disabled performers to overcome the obstacles posed by
theatrical managements failing to consider them on an equal basis with
their able-bodied counterparts, is to form their own companies. The
Theatre of the Disabled and the former National Theatre of the Deaf
were both developed as vehicles to further the talents of handicapped
professional performers. The emergence of the Graeae Theatre
Company is another example that springs to mind, though this was
established with largely amateur actors and the implicit object of
dispelling prejudice against disability. However, so far, the International
Year of Disabled People has thrown up a disappointingly small number
of initiatives of this kind. Of course, there is a view which suggests that
such disabled groups of performers reinforce a ghetto mentality.
However, until current attitudes and misconceptions change, it's difficult
to envisage any immediate prospect for the integration of any but the
most exceptional individuals, except in the less frenetic visual arts field.

Q.   *Both of us appreciate the development of the Shape
organisation and its work in London and other
areas. Can you mention some other schemes which
appear to have merit?*

One of the most exciting initiatives, which I believe is aided by North
West Shape, is the work of the artist Peter Senior in hospitals in
Manchester. This scheme has totally transformed the interiors of some of
the most appallingly drab hospitals.

Another long established project is on North Humberside, where almost half the 4,000 hospital beds are for the mentally impaired. During the period October 1977 to April 1978, Lincolnshire & Humberside Arts, in association with the Humberside Area Health Authority, promoted more than 30 professional arts and crafts events in hospitals for the mentally ill and handicapped in North Humberside. The emphasis was placed on events in which the patients could participate, especially art, crafts, music, puppetry and movement, and the culmination was an exhibition, *From Darkness to Light*, of the art of the mentally handicapped, mounted in Hull. Visits by the EMMA Theatre Company, the Janet Smith Dance Company and the poet Patricia Beer were also funded by the Association at hospitals in the area. The success of the initial scheme led to the provision of funds from the Job Creation Programme and the Priestman Trust to enable professional artists to be appointed by the Association in subsequent years to work in hospitals in the area.

Of course such initiatives demand close co-operation between the artists, patients, hospital staff, hospital authorities and arts funding agencies. More collaborative effort has led Greater London Arts Association, PHAB and Shape to hold a seminar to encourage the development of a shared interest and participation in the arts by the young disabled and able-bodied.

The onset of the International Year of Disabled People has encouraged some professional theatre companies to work with handicapped people, and led others to recognise that disability was a topical theme for their productions. If I single out two particular initiatives, it is simply to illustrate the type of work taking place. The Yorkshire-based company Interplay is involved in a project at high-dependency wards in mental hospitals. Working with eight performers, and slightly more volunteers, they transform the ward environment into a "circus" for a day, establishing one-to-one relationships with patients in the process. Theatre Clywd's Outreach Company has been taking drama into schools in North Wales to create an awareness among the children of the problems of disability. The children are encouraged to imagine what it is like to be disabled, and young volunteers spend half a day in a wheelchair, blindfolded or with immobilised arms and hands as part of the session.

Finally, many handicapped people are unaware of the opportunities that exist for them to attend arts events, or are unclear about the accessibility of venues; disabled artists may want information on employment opportunities in the arts, and local disabled groups may want lists of professional performers willing to entertain them. That is why I particularly welcome the proposal to establish a telephone "help-line" information service in Greater London on arts and disability, with the aid of funds from Capital Radio.

Q. *Despite imaginative ideas in the arts, there appears to be a lack of similar progress to help the disabled through better access to theatres and halls. Would you develop your views about this difficulty?*

Although increasing attention is paid to the needs of the handicapped when new buildings are designed, a physically handicapped person's choice of accessible arts facilities remains very limited. Accessibility to the arts implies the removal of any barrier which excludes sections of the public. These include architectural barriers, such as steps, small or difficult-to-open doors, narrow corridors, inaccessible telephones, restaurants and toilet facilities, and the lack of suitable lifts. Not only are the barriers confined to the auditorium and front of house; if handicapped people are going to be encouraged to perform, consideration must also be given to access to stage and green room.

A challenging report[3] published by the Greater London Arts Association, in conjunction with the Greater London Association for the Disabled, highlighted the many obstacles preventing handicapped people from attending and enjoying arts events. The report was based on research undertaken at 78 venues used for the Greenwich Festival, and it revealed that "roughly half the buildings checked have entrances that are impossible or hazardous for disabled people." Consultations with disabled people in other areas suggests that the result of the survey in Greenwich is fairly representative of the situation in other London boroughs.

Failure on the part of the managements of arts venues to respond to the creation of access opportunities for the handicapped is not intentional, of course; it is usually due to oversight or ignorance of the enormous physical and psychological difficulties which confront the disabled in getting in and around their buildings. In the course of the Silver Jubilee Committee's investigation into improving access for the disabled,[4] it made an informal approach to managers, administrators and leisure service directors to discover their views and experiences about the way in which disabled people could and did use theatres, cinemas, civic halls and other amenities. As the report points out, what access means to managers varies enormously, ranging from a realisation of the need to enter the building and reach a seat or wheelchair space, to a much greater awareness of what disability means, so that thought had been given to parking, lavatories and refreshments as well. Methods used to accommodate the disabled in the most comfortable theatres consisted primarily of making arrangements for the wheelchair-bound; installation of induction loop systems to help people with hearing difficulties, or alterations to benefit the partially sighted, such as painting doors in contrasting colours, have not received anything like the same attention, although they cost comparatively little. Indeed making a building accessible does not necessarily mean making it more expensive. Thoughtful design costs less in the long term and results in facilities which serve all sections of the community. Unfortunately, past experience tends to suggest that if adequate facilities for the disabled are included at the design stage, it is more often due to the initiative of an individual rather than the result of official directives or guidelines.

In an attempt to secure an improvement in access for the disabled to arts centres, concert halls, theatres, cinemas, galleries and museums, a new trust (ACCESS: The National Association of Arts Facilities for Disabled People) is to be established to provide technical advice and, where appropriate, grants to arts buildings throughout the UK wishing to adapt their premises to facilitate access opportunities.

Another encouraging initiative is the working party set up by the UK Committee of the International Year of Disabled People, to examine the information used on public buildings, and in theatre, concert hall and gallery advertising, to denote the facilities available for the disabled. The working party is particularly concerned about the misuse of the well-known wheelchair symbol in publicity, and is anxious that information on facilities for other varieties of handicap, e.g. impaired sight or hearing, is reflected in promotional material and the classified listings of venues in newspapers.

Not all of the obstacles to accessibility are architectural, though. Many of the barriers are attitudinal; fire regulations, insurance liabilities, and preconceived ideas about the safety and desirability of having handicapped people on the premises all serve to inhibit the disabled visitor. Often the disabled person is segregated from the rest of the patrons at the front or rear of the auditorium because of safety regulations; and incidentally, the considerable differences in the interpretation of safety regulations between the various licensing authorities is astonishing.

Until concerted pressure is brought to bear on the authorities, disabled people will remain trapped in a dreadful Catch 22 situation: they are unable to attend arts events, so managers of venues assume there is no demand for entry from the disabled, and make no attempt to remedy deficiencies which prevent easy access, and so no disabled attend.

Councillor A. Walls, Convener of Aberdeen City Art Gallery and Museums committee, has pointed out that "it is not special consideration that disabled people need; it is the ordinary provision made accessible. Once there, they can contribute to and enjoy the 'ordinary' world equally with everyone else. We shall have ended discrimination against disabled people when a wheelchair is no more remarkable in an office, shop, factory, council chamber or museum, than a pair of spectacles."[5] Amen to that.

Q.   *Is the situation in America comparable to Britain or have they made more progress there?*

Despite my quote from *Arts and the Handicapped — An Issue of Access* earlier, the United States of America has shown a far more enlightened concern for the plight of the disadvantaged than we in Britain. To a degree this may have been the direct result of legislation. The Architectural Barriers Act of 1968, for example, requires that any new public building in receipt of government funds, or any facility being adapted or renovated, must be fully accessible to all handicapped persons. Section 504 of the Rehabilitation Act 1973 goes even further in its advocacy for the handicapped when it states that "no otherwise qualified handicapped person in the US . . . shall, solely by reason of his handicap be excluded from participating in, be denied the benefits of, or be subjected to discrimination under any programme or activity receiving federal financial assistance." This means that any public arts facility, theatre, concert hall, arts centre or museum may jeopardise future government aid if it fails to provide accessibility for all to its presentations or premises.

Since 1969, Hospital Audiences Incorporated has arranged for more than 1½ million individuals in hospitals, prisons, nursing homes, drug treatment and prevention centres, and other health and social service settings in New York, to attend different cultural events in places such as Lincoln Centre, Carnegie Hall, Broadway and off-Broadway theatres etc. HAI is the nearest equivalent in the USA to Shape in the UK, though considerably better funded. It has brought hundreds of performed arts events and participatory arts workshop sessions to institutions to develop the creative abilities of those confined there. Over 150,000 individuals benefit annually from HAI services and many cities in the USA now have affiliated branches.

The National Endowment of the Arts has made a commitment towards helping to eliminate the barriers — both physical and social —

which prevent handicapped Americans from enjoying the arts on a regular basis. Over 1% of its budget is directed to institutions concerned with the handicapped and elderly. It supports professional theatre staff working with psychiatric patients in hospitals; arts are brought to the elderly through the NEA's Expansion Arts and Special Projects Schemes; NEA projects provide assistance for the removal of architectural barriers for the physically impaired. The NEA and the Bureau of Prisons have also developed an artist-in-residence programme which has minimised tension among inmates.

Training opportunities in the arts are also more advanced for the handicapped in the United States. The Gallaudet College in Washington, for example, has built up an enviable reputation for its preparation of deaf students for careers in the performing arts. No comparable opportunities are available in the UK; and while such training does not guarantee professional arts employment for students once they have graduated, some at least have the opportunity of work with American dance companies or with the long established National Theatre of the Deaf.

Throughout the USA there are now tactile museums and exhibitions for the visually disabled. The Mary Duke Biddle Gallery at the North Carolina Museum of Art was one of the first tactile galleries for the blind. Three rooms constantly change exhibits—textured walls, tactile sculpture and intensely lit paintings. Everything on display can be touched and examined by the public. The gallery attracts 10,000 visitors a month, only 10% of them visually impaired. "People perhaps come out of curiosity at first, but then they realise that the works are of museum quality," says the Museum's former curator, Maya Reid.[6] She believes the gallery satisfied a great craving to touch among the sighted as well as the blind. As you can imagine, not everyone approves of the "hands-on" approach, either because of the risk of damage to objects in collections, or because the works exhibited are often of inferior quality to those on display elsewhere. So some new facilities, such as the Smithsonian Institute's Air and Space Museum, Washington, while making no attempt to "segregate" the disabled, ensure that most of the exhibits are fully accessible to handicapped visitors. In Britain the Museum's Association has compiled a list of museums with *Facilities for the Blind,*[7] and galleries are increasingly arranging tactile exhibitions.

Of course initiatives in other countries besides the USA may be of interest to practitioners here. That is why the proposed creation of Interlink, an international clearing house to exchange information and experiences between those working in the field of the arts and the handicapped, is a welcome development.

Q.   What action has been taken here about legislation?

Hitherto, unlike the USA, there have been no sanctions against those in Britain who fail to provide suitable facilities for access for the disabled in public buildings. Alf Morris, former Minister for the Disabled, has frequently urged local authorities and others to make greater use of the provisions of the Chronically Sick and Disabled Persons Act 1970 to improve the quality of life for the physically and mentally impaired. One intention of the Act was that the disabled should be able to take advantage of recreation and education opportunities outside their homes in the same way as the able-bodied.

The 1970 legislation stated that:

Any person undertaking the provision of any building or premises to which the public are admitted, whether on payment or otherwise, shall in the means of access both to and within the building or premises, and in the making of parking facilities and sanitary conveniences to be available (if any) make provision, in so far as it is in the circumstances both *practicable and reasonable*, for the needs of the members of the public visiting the building or premises who are disabled.

The problem was the words "practicable and reasonable." They have provided a loophole for those who did not care to abide by the spirit of the Act. Consequently, despite the high aspirations once held for this legislation it has been clear for a long time that the Act had no teeth. So new buildings were frequently erected without adequate facilities.

However, the Disabled Persons (No 2) Bill, currently in the last stages of its passage through Parliament, seeks to remedy this situation. Clause 3 of the Bill deals with the need to improve the legislative framework securing access for disabled people into and out of new public buildings. It makes it mandatory for local planning authorities when granting planning permission to draw the attention of developers to their responsibility under the 1970 Act, and to the *Code of Practice for Access for the Disabled to Buildings*.[8] Moreover, the Bill substitutes the words "appropriate provision" for the phrase in the 1970 Act, "provision, in so far as it is in the circumstances both practicable and reasonable." If, as expected, the Bill receives the Royal Assent, the new clause should increase the access opportunities of the disabled. Unfortunately, because the legislation only applies to new buildings, the problem of inadequate facilities at existing arts venues remains, and sadly local authorities usually regard the adaptation of these to meet the needs of the disabled, as a low priority.

Q. *A final comment?*

In the final analysis social integration and acceptance cannot be simply legislated for. Making the arts accessible to the handicapped is not just a question of providing ramps, special facilities, and more funding. Rather it requires many levels of positive action; removal of architectural barriers, statutory legislation covering existing premises with powers for enforcement, exchange and dissemination of information, and co-operation between the several agencies involved, i.e. Department of Education and Science, the Department of Health and Social Security, the Department of the Environment, arts funding bodies, trusts, RAAs, local authorities and the specialist handicapped organisations. Above all, it requires a radical change of attitude; an end to the many economic and architectural excuses; a greater awareness of the importance of serving this very substantial minority; and a realisation that they are part of, not apart from society.

Rod Fisher is Information Officer for the Arts Council of Great Britain. This interview is based loosely on an article he wrote, which was published in *Municipal Entertainment* in November 1978.

REFERENCES

1. *Arts and the Handicapped — An Issue of Access.* Report from Educational Facilities Laboratories and the National Endowment for the Arts. New York, 1975.
2. *A Case For The Arts.* Paper by Michael Jon Spencer, Executive Director, Hospital Audiences Inc. New York, 1976.
3. *Needing A Push: How The Arts Neglect The Disabled.* Report published by the Greater London Arts Association in conjunction with the Greater London Association for the Disabled, 1979.
4. *Can Disabled People Go Where You Go?* Report of the Silver Jubilee Committee on Improving Access for Disabled People. Published by the Department of Health and Social Security, 1979.
5. *Museums and the Handicapped.* Published by the Leicestershire Museums, Art Galleries and Records and Service for Educational Services in Museums, University of Leicester, 1976.
6. "The Barriers Come Down." Article by Judy Gilliom in *The Cultural Post* (No 14; Nov/Dec 1977); published by the National Endowment for the Arts, Washington DC.
7. *Facilities for the Blind.* A list of museums issued by The Museums Association, 34 Bloomsbury Way, London WC1A 2SF, 1981.
8. *Code of Practice for Access for the Disabled to Buildings.* The British Standards Institution, ref. BS 5810; 1979.

NOTE: A *Reading List on Arts and the Handicapped (Reference Sheet 7)* is available free from the Information and Research Section at the Arts Council of Great Britain, 105 Piccadilly, London W1V 0AU. Requests should be accompanied by a self-addressed label and a postage stamp.

CONTRIBUTORS

LYNN ESKOW, MSc in Education and BA(Drama) of the University of California at Berkeley, has 18 years' experience as a teacher of improvisational drama with children. At the time of her contribution she was Co-ordinator for the British Institute for the Study of the Arts in Therapy, but she has since returned to work in the USA.

ROD FISHER is Information Officer of the Arts Council of Great Britain responsible for liaison over matters concerning arts and the handicapped. He has previously worked in local authority arts and entertainment departments.

CLAUDIA FLANDERS was born in New York City and gained her BA degree in 1954. She married Michael Flanders in 1959 and has two daughters. Since Michael's death in 1975 she has resided in London, engaged in voluntary work with the disabled, and served on the Silver Jubilee Committee concerned with access for the disabled. She is a member of Ealing Community Health Council, the charity Outset, and is Disability Consultant with the National Bus Company.

DOROTHY HEATHCOTE became a Lecturer at the University of Newcastle-upon-Tyne at the age of 24, and is now Senior Lecturer at the School of Education, responsible for teaching drama as education, especially in the Master's degree and advanced Diploma course for teachers.

SUE INNES, who acted as Reporter at the Stirling seminar, is a freelance journalist specialising in the social services, and contributes to *Social Work Today, New Age* and BBC Radio Scotland. She is also a painter.

SUE JENNINGS, DipSocAnthrop, RDTH(Psych), LRAM, LGSM, is Senior Lecturer in Dramatherapy at Hertfordshire College of Art and Design and Adviser to the College of Ripon and York St John course. She is an author and founder-editor of the journal of the British Association of Dramatherapy, and consultant to several education, social service and hospital authorities in Britain and Europe.

PAT KEYSELL trained at the Central School of Speech and Drama, later specialising in mime with Claude Chagrin and Jacques Lecoq. She is a mime artist, the author of *Motives for Mime* based on her teaching experience, and organises the annual Festival of Mime for the National Deaf Children's Society.

JOYCE LAING is a qualified Art Therapist working freelance in psychiatric hospitals and penal institutions. She is chairperson of the Scottish Society of Art and Psychopathology.

GINA LEVETE trained in Ballet, and after nine years' experience using dance movement in classes in prisons and hospitals, she founded "Shape." A Churchill Fellowship allowed her to investigate the role of the arts with the disabled. She has now resigned as Director to write a book on her experiences and aims, and is a freelance tutor.

GEOFFREY LORD qualified as an Associate of the Institute of Bankers and MA in Applied Social Studies. Following experience in teaching and youth work he was a member of the Probation and After-Care Service for 15 years, latterly being Deputy Chief Probation Officer in Greater Manchester, and acting as Director of the Selcare Trust which he helped to found. In 1977 he was appointed Secretary and Treasurer of the Carnegie UK Trust.

DAVID MUMFORD is a trained Mobility Officer with the blind and currently holds a senior position in the Coventry Social Services department with responsibility for services to the visually handicapped. He commenced Drama with the Blind along with two drama tutors, Judy Fairclough and Kate Green.

ALASTAIR PYE qualified as a teacher at Moray House College, Edinburgh, following training at the Royal Scottish Academy of Drama and Music. After a period as Head of Music in a Birmingham comprehensive school, he was appointed the first Music Therapist in special education in the Central Region of Scotland.

BILL SEARY, who acted as a Reporter at the Dartington seminar, is Head of the International Department of the National Council of Voluntary Organisations.

VERONICA SHERBORNE qualified in Physical Education, including physiotherapy, at Bedford College of PE and then trained at the Manchester Studio of Art and Movement under Rudolf Laban. She has taught at the Canadian Child and Youth Drama Association and the Universities of Alberta, Bristol, Rome and Trondheim. She is Senior Lecturer in the Department of Special Education, Bristol Polytechnic, and tutors on courses for Social Workers and teachers including a DES course "Living, Learning and Teaching in areas of longstanding educational disadvantage."

CHERRY VOOGHT holds the Diploma of the Drama Board and is now a Board member, and acts as an Adviser to the National Federation of Women's Institutes on speech and drama. She originated their Effective Speech Courses, is a playwright and has acted as consultant to the BBC.

HENRY WALTON is Professor of Psychiatry at the University of Edinburgh and Chairman of the Scottish Committee on Arts and Disability.

DAVID WARD was trained as a teacher at Trent Park and Matlock Colleges of Education. He has over 12 years' experience as a teacher of music and the education of backward children. From 1968-1976 he was organiser of the action-research project "Music for Slow Learners" sponsored by CUKT and the Standing Conference for Amateur Music at the Dartington College of the Arts where he is a Senior Lecturer.

DIRECTORY OF USEFUL ADDRESSES
OF ORGANISATIONS CONCERNED WITH THE
ARTS AND NEEDS OF THE DISABLED

It is possible to list only the main offices known to the editor and no responsibility is accepted by the editor or publisher for any errors or omissions in the information provided.

The addresses are provided in case an arts group requires a first contact with an organisation representing disability or for a disabled representative wishing to gain knowledge of arts activities.

Arts Councils

Arts Council of Great Britain — 105 Piccadilly, London W1V 0AU
01-629 9495

Arts Council of Northern Ireland — 181a Stranmillis Road,
Belfast BT9 5DU
0232 663591

Scottish Arts Council — 19 Charlotte Square,
Edinburgh EH2 4DF
031-226 6051

Welsh Arts Council — Holst House, 9 Museum Place,
Cardiff CF1 3NX
0222 394711

Regional Arts Associations

East Midlands Arts Association — Mountfields House, Forest Road,
Loughborough,
Leicestershire LE11 3HU
0509 218292

Eastern Arts Association — 8/9 Bridge Street, Cambridge
0223 67707

Greater London Arts Association — 25-31 Tavistock Place,
London WC1H 9SF
01-388 2211

Lincolnshire and Humberside Arts — Saint Hugh's, Newport,
Lincoln LN1 3DN
0522 33555

Merseyside Arts Association — Bluecoat Chambers, School Lane,
Liverpool L1 3BX
051-709 0671/2/3

Northern Arts	10 Osborne Terrace, Newcastle-upon-Tyne NE2 1NZ 0632 816334
North West Arts	12 Harter Street, Manchester M1 6HY 061-228 3062
South East Arts Association	9/10 Crescent Road, Tunbridge Wells, Kent TN2 2LU 0892 41666
Southern Arts Association	19 Southgate Street, Winchester, Hampshire SO23 7EB 0962 55099
South West Arts	23 Southernhay East, Exeter, Devon EX1 1QL 0392 38924
West Midlands Arts	Lloyds Bank Chambers, Market Street, Stafford ST16 2AP 0785 59231
Yorkshire Arts Association	Glyde House, Glydegate, Bradford, West Yorkshire BD5 0BQ 0274 23051
South East Wales Arts Association	Victoria Street, Cwmbran, Gwent NP44 3JP
CRAFTS COUNCIL	12 Waterloo Place, London SW1Y 4AU 01-930 4811

Reference books for addresses include:

The Municipal Year Book ISBN 0305 5906	published by Municipal Publications Ltd 178-202 Great Portland Street London W1N 6NH

Government Departments

Department of Education and Science	Higher and Further Education, Elizabeth House, York Road, London SE1 7PH 01-928 9222
Department of Health and Social Security	Services for Socially Handicapped Division, Alexander Fleming House, Elephant and Castle, London SE1 6BY 01-407 5522
Scottish Office	Social Work Services Group, 43 Jeffrey Street, Edinburgh EH1 3DN 031-556 9233
	Scottish Education Department, Arts and Sport, 113 Rose Street, Edinburgh EH2 3DT 031-226 5016
Welsh Office	Social Work Service, Pearl Assurance House, Greyfriars Road, Cardiff CF1 3RT 0222 44151
	Education Department, Government Buildings, Ty Glas, Llanishen, Cardiff CF4 5PL 0222 753271
Northern Ireland Office	Department of Education, Youth Arts & Libraries, Londonderry House, Chichester Street, Belfast 0232 32253
	Social Work Advisory Group, Dundonald House, Upper Newtownards Road, Belfast BT4 3SF 0232 650111

There are of course several divisions in each government department. The *Civil Service Year Book* lists their officers and responsibilities. Those stated above may be the appropriate first point of inquiry.

Reference books include:

Civil Service Year Book ISBN 0 11 630245 3	published annually by HMSO
Vacher's Parliamentary Companion	published quarterly by A. S. Kerswill Ltd, Leeder House, Erskine Road, London NW3 3AJ

Arts Organisations

It would be unfair to list only a few of the many theatre companies which provide performances and workshops. The appropriate reference book is the *British Alternative Theatre Directory* which lists:

Alternative theatre companies	over 100
Young People's Theatre companies	over 50
Puppet companies	over 90
Arts centres and arts associations	

SHAPE is a registered company and charity which links artists and arts companies with organisations and institutions for the disabled and disadvantaged.

SHAPE	Ms Seona Reid, Director, 7 Fitzroy Square, London W1P 6AE 01-338 9622
Shape in Lincolnshire and Humberside	Lincolnshire & Humberside Arts, St Hugh's, 23 Newport, Lincoln 0522 33555
Shape in the North West	North West Shape, 21 Whalley Road, Whalley Range, Manchester M16 8AD 061-226 9120
Shape up North	The Belle Vue Centre, Belle Vue Road, Leeds LS3 1HG 0532 31005
East Midlands Shape	New Farm, Walton by Kimcote, Nr Lutterworth, Leicestershire LE11 3HU 045-55 3882
West Midlands Region	Art Link, 12 Homesford Terrace, North Street, Newcastle under Lyme, Staffs 0782 614170
Southern Region·	The Other Oxfordshire Theatre, c/o Cowley St Christopher First School, Temple Road, Cowley, Oxford 0865 778119
South West Shape	c/o South West Arts, 23 Southernhay East, Exeter, Devon EX1 1QL 0392 38924
Scottish Committee for Arts and Disability	18/19 Claremont Crescent, Edinburgh EH7 4QD 031-556 3882

Welsh Committee

c/o South East Wales
Arts Association,
Victoria Street, Cwmbran,
Gwent NP44 3JP
06333 67530

The following organisations are listed because they have an additional role and will give advice about arts/craft activities and may provide an information or bulletin service:

Action Space

The Drill Hall, 16 Chenies Street,
London WC1
01-637 7664

Association of Dance Therapists

7 Ashlake Road, Streatham,
London SW16

British Association of Art Therapists

13c Northwood Road,
London N6 5TL

British Association of Drama
Therapists

7 Hatfield Road, St Albans, Herts.

British Society for Music Therapy

48 Lancaster Road, London N6
01-883 1331

British Institute for the Study of the
Arts in Therapy (and Sesame)

Christchurch, 27 Blackfriars Road,
London SE1 8NY
01-633 9690

British Library of Tape Recordings
for Hospital Patients

12 Lant Street, London SE1 1QR
01-407 9417

British Theatre Association

9 Fitzroy Square, London W1P 6AE
01-387 2666

Calibre-Cassette Library for the
Blind and Handicapped

Aylesbury, Bucks HP20 1HU
0296 32339

Central Bureau for Educational
Visits and Exchanges

43 Dorset Street, London W1H 3FN
01-486 5101
and
3 Bruntsfield Crescent,
Edinburgh EH10 4HD
031-447 8024

Cockpit Theatre and Arts Workshop

Gateforth Street, Marylebone,
London NW1
01-262 7907

Council for Music in Hospitals

340 Lower Road, Little Bookham,
Surrey KT23 4RE

The Dance Drama Theatre

1 The Warren, Carshalton Beeches,
Surrey SM5 4EQ
01-643 4833

Drama with the Blind — Advisory Group, c/o Royal National Institute for the Blind, 224/8 Great Portland Street, London S1N 6AA 01-388 1266

The Drama Board and Central Council for Amateur Theatre — PO Box 44, Banbury, Oxon OX15 4EQ 0295 50860

Educational Drama Association — Drama Centre, Reaside School, Rea St South, Birmingham B5 6LB 021-622 3107

Gardens for the Disabled Trust — Headcorn Manor, Headcorn, Kent TN27 9NP 0622 890360

Handicrafts Advisory Association for the Disabled — 103 Brighton Road, Purley CR2 4HD

Inter-Action Trust — Talacre Open Space, 15 Wilkin Street, Kentish Town, London NW5 01-485 0881

Interim Theatre Company Limited (Deaf-Hearing company) — 3 Spring Lane, London SE25 4SP 01-656 9653/4

Interplay Trust — Hall Lane Community Centre, 65 Hall Lane, Armley, Leeds LS12 1 PQ 0532 634380

Ludus Dance in Education — Rhodes House, 114 St Leonardgate, Lancaster LA1 1NN 0524 67728

Minority Arts Advisory Service — 91 Mortimer Street, London W1N 7TA 01-580 1534

National Association for Drama in Education and Children's Theatre, and National Council of Theatre for Young People — c/o British Theatre Centre, 9 Fitzroy Square, London W1P 6AE 01-387 2666

National Listening Library (Talking Books for the Handicapped) — 49 Great Cumberland Place, London W1H 7LH 01-723 5008

National Operatic and Dramatic Association — 1 Crestfield Street, London WC1H 8AU 01-837 5655

Natural Dance Theatre — The Natural Dance Workshop, Playspace, Peto Place, London NW1 4DT 01-935 1410

Neighbourhood Open Workshops   2-4 University Road, Belfast BT7 1NT
0232 42910

Nordoff Music Therapy Centre   c/o Goldie Leigh Hospital,
Lodge Hill,
Abbey Wood, London SE2 0AY

Partially Sighted Society
(Large Print Music scheme)   40 Wordsworth Street, Hove,
East Sussex BN3 5BH
0273 736053

Polka Children's Theatre   240 The Broadway, Wimbledon,
London SW19 1SB
01-542 4258

Puppet Centre—Educational
Puppetry Association   c/o Battersea Arts Centre,
Lavender Hill, London SW11 5TJ
01-223 5356

Royal School of Needlework   25 Princes Gate, London SW7 1QE
01-589 0077

Scottish Mime Theatre   36a Lauriston Place,
Edinburgh EH3 9EZ
031-229 2821

Standing Conference for
Amateur Music   26 Bedford Square,
London WC1B 3HU
01-636 4066

Scottish Amateur Music Association   7 Randolph Crescent,
Edinburgh EH3 7TH

Tibble Trust (Music for the Elderly)   36 Belsize Court, Wedderburn,
London NW3 5QJ

Ulverscroft Large Print Book Ltd   The Green, Bradgate Road, Anstey,
Leicester LE7 7FW
053-721 4325

Wireless for the Bedridden   81b Corbets Tey Road, Upminster,
London
04022 50051

The Workshop, Edinburgh   34 Hamilton Place,
Edinburgh EH3 5AX
031-225 7942

Reference books for addresses include:
British Alternative Theatre Directory
ISBN 0 903931 19 2   John Offord Publications Ltd,
PO Box 64, Eastbourne BN21 3LW
Directory of Arts Centres 2   John Offord Publications Ltd
(as above)
available also from:
Arts Council Shop, 8 Long Acre,
Covent Garden, London WC2E 9LG

Children's World of Art
(A directory of Children's Arts
Activities)

Central Bureau of Educational Visits
and Exchanges,
Seymour Mews House,
Seymour Mews, London W1
01-486 5101
or
International Year of the Child Trust,
8 Wakley Street, London EC1

Community Arts Merseyside

Merseyside Arts Association,
6 Bluecoat Chambers, School Lane,
Liverpool L1 3BX
051-709 0671

Contacts
(Annual magazine listing TV, Stage,
Screen and Radio contacts)

The Spotlight, 42-43 Cranbourn Street,
London WC2H 7AP
01-437 7631

ORGANISATIONS with a responsibility and concern for the disabled or
disadvantaged with knowledge of arts and crafts activities:

Councils for Disability and Social Service

Royal Association for Disability
and Rehabilitation

25 Mortimer Street,
London W1N 8AB
01-637 5400

Northern Ireland Committee for
the Handicapped and NI Council
of Social Service

2 Annadale Avenue, Belfast BT7 3JH
0232 640011

Scottish Council on Disability and
Scottish Council of Social Service

18/19 Claremont Crescent,
Edinburgh EH7 4QD
031-556 3882

Wales Council for the Disabled and
Council of Social Service for Wales

Llys Ifor, Crescent Road,
Caerphilly CF8 1XL
0222 869224

National Council for Voluntary
Organisations

26 Bedford Square,
London WC1B 3HU
01-636 4066

Other Organisations

AFASIC— Association for All
Speech Impaired Children

347 Central Markets, Smithfield,
London EC1A 9NH
01-236 6487

Barnardo's

Tanners Lane, Barkingside, Ilford,
Essex IG6 1QG
01-550 8822

Barnardo's, Scotland	22 Drumsheugh Gardens, Edinburgh EH3 7RP 031-226 5241
Breakthrough Trust (for the deaf and hearing)	66/68 Greenwich South Street, London SE10 8UN 01-691 6229
British Association of Social Workers	16 Kent Street, Birmingham 5 021-622 3911
Centre for Studies in Mental Handicap	c/o Gogarburn Hospital, Edinburgh EH12 9BJ 031-339 4242
Cruse (the national organisation for the widowed and their children)	Cruse House, 126 Sheen Road, Richmond, Surrey TW9 1UR 01-940 4818
Disabilities Studies Unit	Dr Duncan Guthrie, Wildhanger, Amberley, Arundel, W Sussex BN18 9NR
Disabled Living Foundation	Miss D. Kennard, Music Officer, 346 Kensington High Street, London W14 8NS 01-602 2491
Gingerbread	35 Wellington Street, London WC2 01-240 0953
Invalid Children's Aid Association	126 Buckingham Palace Road, London SW1W 9SB 01-730 9891
King's Fund Centre	126 Albert Street, London NW1 7NF 01-267 6111
Learning Disabilities Unit	Mr C. Stephenson, Department of Education, The University of Southampton, SO9 5NH 0703 559122
MIND — National Association for Mental Health	22 Harley Street, London W1N 2ED 01-637 0741
National Bureau for Handicapped Students	40 Brunswick Square, London WC1N 1AZ 01-278 3127
National Children's Bureau	8 Wakley Street, Islington, London EC7V 7QE 01-278 9441
National Council for One Parent Families	255 Kentish Town Road, London NW5 2LX 01-267 1361

National Deaf Children's Society	31 Gloucester Place, London W1H 4EA 01-486 3251
National Federation of Gateway Clubs, *and* National Society for Mentally Handicapped Children and Adults	117-123 Golden Lane, London EC1Y 0RT 01-253 9433
National Federation of Women's Institutes	39 Eccleston Street, London SW1W 9NT 01-730 7212
National Institute of Adult Education (England and Wales)	19b De Montfort Street, Leicester LE1 7GE 0533 538977
National Society for Autistic Children	1a Golders Green, London NW11 8EA 01-458 4375
National Union of Townswomen's Guilds	2 Cromwell Place, London SW7 2JG 01-589 8817
Partially Sighted Society	40 Wordsworth Street, Hove, East Sussex BN3 5BH 0273 736053
PHAB – Physically Handicapped and Able Bodied	42 Devonshire Street, London W1N 1LN 01-637 7475
Royal National Institute for the Blind	Sports and Recreation Officer, 224/8 Great Portland Street, London W1N 6AA 01-388 1266
Royal National Institute for the Deaf	105 Gower Street, London WC1E 6AH 01-387 8033
Scottish Association for Mental Health	Ainslie House, 11 St Colme Street, Edinburgh EH3 6AG 031-225 3062
Scottish Association for the Deaf	Moray House, Edinburgh EH8 8AQ 031-556 8137
Scottish Community Education Centre	4 Queensferry Street, Edinburgh EH2 4PA 031-225 9451
Scottish Council for Single Parents	44 Albany Street, Edinburgh EH1 3QR 031-556 3899
Scottish Council for Spastics	Rhuemore, 22 Corstorphine Road, Edinburgh EH12 6HP 031-337 9876

Scottish Institute for Adult
Education

4 Queensferry Street,
Edinburgh EH2 4PA
031-226 5404

Scottish Society for Autistic Children

1st Floor, 12 Picardy Place,
Edinburgh EH1 3JT
031-552 8459

Scottish Society for the Mentally
Handicapped

13 Elmbank Street, Glasgow G2 4QA
041-226 4541

Spastics Society

Recreation Services, 12 Park Crescent,
London W1N 4EQ
01-636 5020

Volunteer Centre

29 Lower King's Road,
Berkhamsted, Herts HP4 2AB
04427 73311

Widows Advisory Trust – National
Association of Widows

c/o Stafford District Voluntary
Service Centre, Chell Road,
Stafford ST16 2QA
0785 45465

Reference books for addresses include:

*ABC of services and information
for disabled people*

Disablement Income Group,
Attlee House, Toynbee Hall,
28 Commercial Street,
London E1 6LE

Charities Digest

published annually by the
Family Welfare Association,
501-503 Kingsland Road,
London E8 4AU

Directory for the Disabled

published by
Woodhead Faulkner Ltd,
8 Market Passage, Cambridge

Social Services Year Book
ISBN 0 900313 67 6

published annually by Councils
and Education Press Ltd,
42 Great Portland Street,
London W1N 5AH

Voluntary Social Services
ISBN 0 7199 0956 2

published as a directory of
national organisations by
Bedford Square Press (of NCVO),
26 Bedford Square,
London WC1B 3HU

Year Book of Adult Education

a guide listing all sources of
support for adult education and
colleges from National Institute of
Adult Education,
19b De Montfort Street,
Leicester LE1 7GE

Scottish Directory of Community Education, Community Work and Related Fields

published by Scottish Community Education Centre,
4 Queensferry Street,
Edinburgh EH2 4PA
031-225 9451

FOUNDATIONS operating nationally with an interest in arts and disabilities:

Readers wishing to apply to Foundations are advised to consult the current *Directory of Grant-Making Trusts* for advice about an appropriate form of application and the details of policies of the Foundation. Most Foundations will issue a guideline of policies or give information in response to a preliminary inquiry in preference to the receipt of duplicated or general appeals. If in doubt address letters to the Secretary.

Arts Council Special Trust Fund — Arts Council of Great Britain, 105 Piccadilly, London W1V 0AU

Baring Foundation — 88 Leadenhall Street, London EC3A 3DT

Carnegie United Kingdom Trust — Comely Park House, Dunfermline, Fife KY12 7EJ

Charities Aid Foundation — 48 Pembury Road, Tonbridge, Kent TN9 2JD

Chase Charity — 10 Barley Mow Passage, Chiswick, London W4 4PH

Ernest Cook Trust — Estate Office, Fairford Park, Fairford, Gloucestershire GL7 4JH

Hayward Foundation — 16 Grosvenor Place, London SW1X 7HH

Hilden Charitable Fund — Gort Lodge, Sudbrook Lane, Richmond, Surrey TW10 7AY

Allen Lane Foundation — 32 Chestnut Road, London SE27 9LF

Mount Trust — c/o Pothecary & Barratt, Solicitors, Talbot House, Talbot Court, Gracechurch Street, London EC3V 0BS

Pilgrim Trust — Fielden House, Little College Street, London SW1P 3SH

J. Arthur Rank Group Charity — 12 Warwick Square, London SW1V 2AA

Rayne Foundation — Carlton House, 33 Robert Adam Street, London W1M 5AH

Joseph Rowntree Memorial Trust — Beverley House, Shipton Road, York YO3 6RB

Royal Jubilee Trusts — 8 Buckingham Street, London WC2N 6BU

Sembal Trust — 12 Park Crescent, London W1N 4EQ

Wates Foundation	1260 London Road, London SW16 4EG
Marks & Spencer Ltd	Charity and Community Involvement Dept., Michael House, Baker Street, London W1A 1DN

OTHER FOUNDATIONS with general charitable purposes with an income annually over £100,000:

Alexandra Rose Day	1 Castlenau, Barnes, London SW13 9RP
Bronte Charitable Trust	The Barbinder Trust, Abacus House, Gutter Lane, Cheapside, London EC2V 8AH
C & A Charitable Trust	1 Serjeants' Inn, London EC4Y 1JD
Edward Cadbury Charitable Trust	Elmfield College Walk, Birmingham B29 6LE
Charles Clore Foundation	2 Serjeants' Inn, London EC4Y 1LT
Dowty Group Charitable Trust	Arle Court, Cheltenham, Gloucestershire GL51 0TP
Gatsby Charitable Foundation	13 New Row, St Martin's Lane, London WC2N 4LF
Leon and Bertha Gradel Trust	St Ann's House, St Ann's Place, Manchester, Greater Manchester M2 7LP
Grocers' Charity	Grocers' Hall, Princes Street, London EC2R 8AQ
Hedley Foundation Ltd	Dowgate Hill House, London EC4
Philip Henman Trust	Hayburn House, 80a The Street, Ashtead, Surrey
Dawn James Charitable Foundation	Minister House (Ground Floor), 27 Baldwin Street, Bristol, Avon BS1 1LZ
Ivy Judah Philanthropic Trust	Rex House, 4-12 Regent Street, London SW1
Ernest Kleinwort Charitable Trust Sir Cyril Kleinwort Charitable Settlement	c/o Kleinwort Benson Ltd, 20 Fenchurch Street, London EC3P 3DB
Kennedy Leigh Charitable Trust	"Dane Court," The Bishop's Avenue, London N2
Linbury Trust	13 New Row, St Martin's Lane, London WC2N 4LF
Litchfield Trust	4 King's Arms Yard, Moorgate, London EC2R 7AX

Joseph Lucas Charitable Trust Limited	Lucas Industries Ltd, Great King Street, Birmingham, West Midlands B19 2XF
Manifold Charitable Trust	21 Dean's Yard, London SW1P 3PA
Marble Arch Charitable Trust	Hesketh House, Portman Square, London W1A 4SU
Simon Marks Charitable Trust Miriam Marks Charitable Trust	311 Ballards Lane, London N12 8LZ
Monument Trust	13 New Row, St Martin's Lane, London WC2N 4LF
Moorgate Trust Fund New Moorgate Trust Fund	1 South Audley Street, London W1Y 6JS
Austin and Hope Pilkington Trust	66 St Mary's Butts, Reading RG1 2LG
Joseph Rank Benevolent Trusts	51 London Road, Reigate, Surrey
Rhodes Trust – Public Purposes Fund	Rhodes House, Oxford, Oxfordshire
J. B. Rubens Foundation	Berkeley Square House, Berkeley Square, London W1
Harry and Abe Sherman Foundation	Sherman Group, St David's House, Wood Street, Cardiff CF1 1UX
Barnett Shine Charitable Foundation	Bouverie House, 154 Fleet Street, London EC4
Lily and Marcus Sieff Charitable Foundation	311 Ballards Lane, London N12 8LZ
Sobell Foundation	190 Fleet Street, London EC4A 2AP
Bernard Sunley Charitable Foundation	25 Berkeley Square, London W1A 4AX
Truedene Co. Ltd	13-17 New Burlington Place, London W1
29th May 1961 Charity	Dowgate Hill House, London EC4R 2SY
Vandervell Foundation	9 Cheapside, London EC2V 6AD
Bernard Van Leer Foundation UK Trust	13-17 Old Broad Street, London EC2N 1DL
Maurice Wohl Charitable Trust	9 Cavendish Square, London W1M 0JT

Reference books for addresses include:
The Directory of Grant-Making Trusts
ISBN 0 904757 02 1
published by the Charities Aid Foundation, 48 Pembury Road, Tonbridge, Kent TN9 2JD

Music Competitions Awards and Scholarships	Arts Council of Great Britain, Music Department, 105 Piccadilly, London W1V 0AU
Educational Charities — A Guide to Educational Trust Funds ISBN 0 906252 08 3	National Union of Students (now out of print)
Directory of Scottish Trusts	Edinburgh Council of Social Service, 11 St Colme Street, Edinburgh EH3 6AG New national Directory to be published by the Scottish Council of Social Service
Charities Digest	published by The Family Welfare Association, 501-505 Kingsland Road, Dalston, London E8 4AU
The Grants Register ISBN 0333 23415 4 (for professional and advanced vocational training)	The Macmillan Press Ltd, London
The International Foundation Directory ISBN 0 905118 41 3	Europa Publications Ltd, 18 Bedford Square, London WC1B 3JA
Raising Money from Trusts, etc series of publications	Directory of Social Change, 9 Mansfield Place, London NW3
Guide to Awards and Schemes	Arts Council Shop, 8 Long Acre, Covent Garden, London WC2E 9LG
Fund Raising for and by Small Groups of Volunteers	by T. W. Cynog-Jones, published by The Volunteer Centre, 29 Lower King's Road, Berkhamsted, Herts HP4 2AB
The Give and Take of Sponsorship	published by Commercial Relations Department (Dept D), English Tourist Board, 4 Grosvenor Gardens, London SW1N 0DU